HURT

THE INSPIRING, UNTOLD STORY OF TRAUMA CARE

CATHERINE MUSEMECHE, MD

ForeEdge

An imprint of University Press of New England

www.upne.com

Manufactured in the United States of America

Designed by Eric M. Brooks

Typeset in Fresco by Passumpsic Publishing

For permission to reproduce any of the material in this book,
contact Permissions, University Press of New England, One Court
Street, Suite 250, Lebanon NH 03766; or visit www.upne.com

The names and characteristics of any patients known
to the author have been changed to protect their privacy.
Any resulting resemblance to other persons, living or dead,
is entirely coincidental and unintentional.

Library of Congress Cataloging-in-Publication Data

Names: Musemeche, Catherine, author.

Title: Hurt: the inspiring, untold story of trauma care /
    Catherine Musemeche.

Description: Lebanon, NH: ForeEdge, [2016] | Includes
    bibliographical references and index.

Identifiers: LCCN 2016012430 (print) | LCCN 2016013056 (ebook) |
    ISBN 9781611687965 (cloth) | ISBN 9781611689921 (epub, mobi
    & pdf)

Subjects: MESH: Emergency Medicine—history | Wounds and
    Injuries | Emergency Medical Services—history

Classification: LCC RD93 (print) | LCC RD93 (ebook) |
    NLM WB 105 | DDC 617.1—dc23

LC record available at http://lccn.loc.gov/2016012430

5 4 3 2 1

FOR FIRST RESPONDERS EVERYWHERE,
the brave men and women who risk their lives
every day to save ours

CONTENTS

HURT

INTRODUCTION

INJURIES ARE A PART of daily life that we will never escape. Seemingly random, they come out of nowhere and change our lives. There is no vaccination for injuries and no medicine that will cure us of them either. Once we get hurt, we have to suffer through the healing process, aided by the skillful hands of surgeons who close holes, remove damaged organs, and piece together what remains.

From the national tragedy of a mass shooting to the heartbreak of a local drunk-driving fatality, trauma touches all our lives. It is a disease of epidemic proportions leading to the hospitalization of 2.8 million people every year and the death of approximately 180,000. Injuries are the leading cause of disability for those under the age of sixty-five. The leading killer of children and teenagers, injury preys on the young.

We take for granted that no matter how or where we are injured, someone will call 9-1-1 and trained first responders will show up to insert IVs, stop the bleeding, and swiftly deliver us to a hospital manned by doctors and nurses with the necessary trauma expertise to save our lives.

But it was not always that way.

Our current emergency medical services (EMS) system evolved by fits and starts in pockets of this country where passionate innovators led the way, insisting on better care for the injured for one reason—because it saved lives.

Hurt: The Inspiring, Untold Story of Trauma Care is the story of how trauma care evolved into the effective system that it is today and the dedicated men and women who helped build it. There were crusaders like Dr. James Styner, who, after witnessing the substandard care his family received in a rural emergency room, vowed to change how doctors were trained in trauma care and did. Dr. R Adams Cowley taught us how critical time was to survival and created the Maryland Shock Trauma Hospital, which continues to save thousands of lives a year. Public health expert Sue Baker, believing that injuries could be prevented if we looked hard enough for their cause, culled data from the Baltimore medical examiner's office that led to the first infant car seat legislation.

Some of our most valuable lessons in caring for the injured came out of war—the grassy fields of the Civil War, the trenches of two world wars, the jungles of Vietnam, and the deserts of Iraq and Afghanistan. We owe an immeasurable debt of gratitude not only to the physicians, nurses, and medics who served our country in combat but also to the wounded servicemen and -women from whom we learned lessons that could not have come any other way.

One need look no further than the Boston Marathon bombings of 2013 to appreciate the fact that trauma systems save lives. On April 15, 2013, the day of the bombings, Level I trauma centers (the highest level of expertise) at six area teaching hospitals in Boston treated 264 patients, many with serious injuries. Everyone who made it to the hospital that day survived.

ONE >>

TRANSPORT

1 » ALONG FOR THE RIDE

BY THE TIME we'd arranged to transfer Mr. X to a larger nearby hospital, his wife had already died in our emergency room.

Mr. X's stretcher had come banging through the steel double doors first, brought in by ambulance after a train had hit their stalled car. He was propped up in a sitting position and breathing in deeply, as though he couldn't get enough air. Blood was streaked across his face like war paint, and he was groaning loudly.

"Ambulance!" I called down the hall to the charge nurse.

But as soon as I did, the doors banged open again and there was Mrs. X lying flat and still. Nurse Jenkins, a blur of white streaking around the corner of the tiled hallway, grabbed the foot of the stretcher and led it to our largest room, where we put on casts. It wasn't called a trauma room, but it was understood that if a lot of people needed to crowd in, along with an X-ray machine the size of an oven, that was the only room that would allow it.

"Go get the doctor," Nurse Jenkins said as she grabbed the oxygen mask off the wall and slapped on the EKG leads.

I found Dr. Sanchez in an exam room. "Room 1," I said. "Nurse Jenkins needs you right away."

It was 1976, the summer after my first year of college. Each day I put on my short white coat, name badge, and stethoscope and drove my maroon Ford Pinto to a fifty-bed community hospital in Orange, Texas. I worked at the triage desk, the front lines. Mine was the first set of eyes on patients when they came through the door. I wrote down their complaints, counted their respirations, and took their pulse and blood pressure.

Every day brought new revelations.

I unwrapped blood-soaked dishtowels concealing lacerations of all depths and dimensions on hands and feet. I would lift them gingerly out of their swaddling cocoons and dunk them in stainless steel pans of dilute Betadine. I guided teenagers doubled over by appendicitis to stretchers, helped them get up, and left them with a pink plastic basin to throw up in. I wheeled middle-aged men down the hall for EKGs while they clutched their sweaty chests and called out for their wives.

A continuous stream of people came through those doors, a cross-section of our town—poor, middle class, the rare well-dressed businessman, all shades of skin tone and demeanor. Everyone that passed through that dimly lit hallway was seeking relief from disease, injury, and worry, and most of them found it.

But not all.

There were those we couldn't fix, like the drunk twenty-year-old who dove headfirst into shallow water, severing his spinal cord when his head plowed into the sandy bottom. He was still smiling and flirting when he arrived, intoxicated and unaware that he would never again move his legs. As the gravity of his injury unfolded, he sobered up. Maybe it was our faces that gave it away. No one ever said, "This is it. You'll never party at Cow Creek again." But that's exactly what everyone was thinking.

There was the pregnant woman with a skyrocketing blood pressure who was carried in seizing and foaming at the mouth from preeclampsia. The doctor rushed in with a 60 cc syringe of magnesium sulfate and pushed it into her IV tubing as fast as it would flow, but in a matter of minutes, before he could get all of the lifesaving drug in, her pupils became dilated and fixed, a casualty of a presumed stroke. The damage was done; neither she nor the baby lived.

I soon came to realize how easy it was to lose a life in the split second when a decision must be made and action taken. Sometimes, before you ever laid eyes on a person, that moment had passed. Other times it was staring you in the face, daring you to act. If you were lucky, instinct took over and guided your every move.

The train wreck victims were brought in on a busy Sunday afternoon when all the metal folding chairs were occupied by sunburns, sprained ankles, sore throats, and earaches. Every room was taken, and the brown-tiled hallways were lined with patients.

Dr. Sanchez was the sole physician manning the ER that day. An internist, he was trained to solve problems in a methodical fashion. He questioned patients in excruciating detail and examined them from head to toe. He went back and forth to the radiology department, compulsively viewing X-rays over and over. He struggled to make decisions, and that meant everything took longer than it needed to.

Sometimes the wait was too much for the patients. They would motion me over when they'd had enough. "We'll just check in with our doctor tomorrow," they'd say as they picked up their things and walked off.

Mrs. X's breathing was slow and labored by the time Dr. Sanchez walked in. Nurses swarmed the stretcher, waiting to be told what to do. But there was only one doctor, and everything depended on what he did next. He was still straining to find breath sounds in Mrs. X's now silent chest when Nurse Jenkins slapped a breathing tube into his hand. Then he knew: Mrs. X wasn't going to keep while he was conducting a complete history and physical and looking at two views of the chest. She needed the tube now.

He pried Mrs. X's mouth open with the laryngoscope and looked in. He rocked the blade back and forth. He searched like he was trying to find someone in the top row of the stadium bleachers. He squinted, he grimaced, and just when it looked like he might never find it, a glimmer of recognition registered on his brow and he coaxed the tube into the trachea. Nurse Jenkins attached the ventilation bag and squeezed air into Mrs. X's stiff lungs, but it had all been too much for her by then—the wreck, the delay, and some devastating injury we would never know by name. She could not be revived. Dr. Sanchez pronounced her dead and left to find her husband.

By this time, Mr. X's breathing had turned fast and shallow, and he was moaning. His chest had been crushed between the steering wheel and the front seat, cracking ribs on both sides. When he tried to breathe in, the midportion of his unhinged rib cage floated dangerously free and sharp shards of bone stabbed his lungs. Dr. Sanchez inserted a breathing tube and put Mr. X on a ventilator, hoping this would be enough to stabilize him, but his oxygen levels dropped further with each blood draw. He couldn't survive if they got much lower.

THE TREATMENT OF THE severely injured is a world of its own. What sets trauma apart from almost any other affliction known to mankind is the small window of opportunity, the "golden hour," during which critical action must be taken to save a life. Miss that window and a person who might have gone on to live another twenty, fifty, or even eighty years tragically loses out on that future; likewise, his family, friends, and coworkers are robbed of the chance to share those years.

There are only so many ways to die suddenly from injury—an airway that abruptly closes off, uncontrollable hemorrhage (either external or internal), a heart compressed by air escaping from a collapsed lung, a brain so swollen it can no longer prod a body to breathe. These are the fatal interruptions in the circuitry of life that can kill people before anyone has even thought to call 9-1-1. When your patient dies from one of these mechanisms, unsettling questions emerge. What would we do differently next time? Was this a preventable death? Could we have intervened earlier and changed the outcome? Or was this a death that would get recorded in the "unavoidable" column no matter what we did, the damage judged catastrophic and beyond our means to repair? As trauma medicine improved through the decades, the answers continued to evolve transforming yesterday's fatalities into tomorrow's saves.

The military deserves much of the credit for the miracles that trauma surgeons are able to pull off on a daily basis. Servicemen and -women have rewarded us not only with their bravery but also with what we have been able to learn in treating their injuries.

From the Civil War up through the wars in Iraq and Afghanistan, there has been no better incubator for discovery and innovation than war because of the numbers of wounded and the severity of their injuries. Combat has motivated exponential leaps in every phase of treatment, from prehospital evacuation and stabilization, to in-hospital application of operative tools and techniques, to the third phase of medical care, rehabilitation, where both brain and body are retrained.

On America's own city streets and highways, trauma inevitably intruded on civilian lives as an ever-increasing number of automobiles crowded the roads. The fact that injury was a substantial public health threat jolted the nation's consciousness when the 1966 report *Accidental Death and Disability: The Neglected Disease of Modern Society* was published by the National Academy of Sciences. It opened with the stunning revelation that in 1965 "52 million accidental injuries killed 107,000, temporarily disabled over 10 million, and permanently impaired 400,000 American citizens at a cost of approximately $18 billion."[1] Accidents were cited as the leading cause of death from ages one to thirty-seven and the fourth leading cause of death at all ages.

Deaths from car crashes had been steadily rising each year from 1955 to 1965 thanks to a rapidly expanding interstate highway system coupled with cars that lacked even basic safety features. More people were dying per year from car crashes than had died in the entire Korean War. Equally disturbing were the findings that the nation lacked quality emergency care, especially in the prehospital phase. In an era where there were no recognized standards for EMS and no 9-1-1, transport of the injured to hospitals was disorganized, inefficient, and haphazard.

Accidental Death and Disability served as a blaring call to action for a public health problem that had seemingly snuck up on the American people. The report also laid out a blueprint for how to corral the injury epidemic and improve prehospital response. The report recommended research and education in accident prevention, the development of safety standards, and training the lay public in basic and advanced first aid. It advocated for adopting minimal personnel and equipment standards for ambulance services, including piloting helicopter ambulances. It urged better communication between ambulances in the field and doctors in receiving hospitals.

In 1966, in his State of the Union Address, President Lyndon B. Johnson proposed new safety legislation and the formation of a new executive agency, the Department of Transportation.[2] Johnson had long advocated for highway safety, dating back to his days in the U.S. Senate.

On September 9, 1966, Congress passed two bills—the National Traffic and Motor Vehicle Safety Act, which called for the development of federal vehicle safety standards that would start with 1968 car models, and the Highway Safety Act, which set up a national framework for state highway safety programs and established the Department of Transportation to facilitate traffic safety programs and the development of EMS. The president's remarks at the bill's signing highlighted the urgency of the problem:

> Over the Labor Day weekend, 29 American servicemen died in Vietnam. During the same Labor Day Weekend, 614 Ameri-

cans died on our highways in automobile accidents. . . . Every 11 minutes a citizen is killed on the road. Every day 9,000 are killed or injured—9,000! Last year 50,000 were killed. And the tragic totals have mounted every year. . . . And if our accident rate continues, one out of every two Americans can look forward to being injured by a car during his lifetime. . . .

For years now, we have spent millions of dollars to understand and to fight polio and other childhood diseases. Yet up until now we have tolerated a raging epidemic of highway death—which has killed more of our youth than all other diseases combined.[3]

While these bills got safety programs off the ground, they could not address and fund all the improvements necessary in every state. The 1960s saw improvements in EMS services, but they were spotty and inconsistent from one locale to another. State and federal governments, for the most part, failed to dedicate sufficient resources.

In other words, the furor of injury died down, as it always does when another crisis, such as the Vietnam War, steals the headlines and diverts our attention. The automobile lobby dug in to fight attempts to mandate safety features, fearing the increased costs that would be passed on to consumers. And we citizens kept driving drunk, defied speed limits, and neglected to buckle our seat belts once we finally got them.

And the carnage continued.

For much of the next two decades, it would be left to individual physician leaders, private foundations, medical schools, and municipalities to take the lead in EMS and trauma care. Injury prevention measures were challenged in debates over who was going to underwrite the cost of a safer world. And it would be several more decades before our country had anything close to a national network of trauma care.

But individual heroes, radical thinkers who knew we could

do better and dared to offer solutions, came forward with ideas that would prove to be game changers in trauma care. One such paradigm-shifting advance was born not from research conducted in the halls of academia, but in the middle of the night in a cornfield in Nebraska.

AT 6 P.M. ON FEBRUARY 17, 1976, Dr. James Styner, an orthopedic surgeon from Lincoln, Nebraska, was at the controls of a Beechcraft Barron twin-engine airplane flying his family home from a wedding in Los Angeles, California. As he entered Nebraska airspace around dusk Styner was fatigued, having been at the controls for five hours. Flying in the dark without the assistance of instrument navigation, he encountered a thin cloud layer that forced him to fly at a lower altitude than planned. He became disoriented, lost altitude, and struggled to maintain control of the aircraft as it swooped over a pond, clipped treetops, and came to rest in a field.[4]

His entire family was aboard, including his wife in the front seat next to him and his four children, ranging in age from three to ten years old, in the rear passenger compartment. On the way down, Styner watched helplessly as his wife was struck in the head with a shrapnel-like chunk of propeller that had broken off. The plane came to rest on its side with the wings sheared off and a large hole in the fuselage.

Styner had facial lacerations, a handful of fractured ribs, and a broken shoulder, but he could still move. When he looked around, he realized that his wife had been thrown from the plane on impact. He then checked on his four children. At first glance he could tell they were all alive, but three were unconscious from serious closed head injuries; two of those three would be in a coma for a week. One child's leg was trapped under the fuselage, pinned under a sharp piece of metal. His oldest son was alert but had a broken arm.

Styner stumbled in the dark and after three attempts finally found his wife and confirmed that she was dead. He would check three more times during the night to be sure he hadn't missed any signs that she was still alive, but the verdict remained unchanged. With the temperature dropping (eventually down to 26 degrees F), Styner made a shelter for his children and waited for help to arrive. He waited six long hours with no rescue in sight and was forced to hobble his way to a highway just over half a mile away, where he managed to flag down a car. Two men drove him back to the accident site and helped him load his kids and drove them all to a nearby community hospital.

When they arrived, the rear emergency room door was locked, and they had to wait outside until a night nurse heard them beating on the door and let them in. By this time Styner was having severe chest and shoulder pain and three of his kids were in critical condition, but, incredibly, the nurse would not start any treatment, not even an IV, until two general practitioners from a nearby farm community had arrived.

Already frustrated by the long wait, Styner was stunned when he saw one of the doctors pick up his eight-year-old son and carry him to the X-ray department without supporting his head or stabilizing his neck. Agitated and combative, the child had unmistakable signs of a head injury, a condition that could easily be coupled with a broken neck.

Styner was dazed, in pain, and exhausted, but none of that could mask how dismayed he was by the sluggish and reckless care. He'd seen enough of the trauma care in Podunk, U.S.A. Fearing what might happen next, he called one of his partners in Lincoln, Nebraska, and made arrangements for the Lincoln Air National Guard to transport his family to Lincoln General Hospital, where the emergency room was not only open but also fully staffed with specialists—an emergency room physician, a general surgeon, and a plastic surgeon. As soon as Styner's family arrived, the team "acted like a coiled spring that had been released," he recalled later; they immediately assessed and treated the injured family in an orderly and systematic manner.

For the next year, Styner focused on healing his physical and emotional trauma and getting his family healthy. But he found himself returning to that night and repeatedly relating to his colleagues what had happened to him at that first rural hospital. The nightmare scenario he lived through continued to eat at him: that there had been no system in place to respond to the needs of rural accident victims and that he was left at the mercy of physicians with little to no trauma experience who were fumbling the ball.

"When I can provide better care in the field with limited resources than what my children and I received at the primary care facility, there is something wrong with the system and the system has to be changed," Styner said.[5]

This statement would become a rallying cry as Styner enlisted the help of Dr. Ron Craig, the emergency room physician who had treated him at Lincoln General Hospital that night, to help turn his bitter experience into a way to forever change the care of trauma patients. They came up with the idea of modeling a course for trauma on the Advanced Cardiac Life Support course, which another Lincoln physician, cardiac surgeon Dr. Steve Carveth, had helped to develop in 1975.[6] Styner, Craig, and Jodie Bechtel, a mobile heart team nurse, decided to adopt a similar format and call it Advanced Trauma Life Support (ATLS). The initial goal of the course was to teach physicians working in small community hospitals basic trauma care, including how to diagnose the most imminent threats to life and teach them the skills to treat and avert them.

What made ATLS a game changer was the idea of shaking up the traditional medical model for assessing a patient that required conducting an exhaustive history and physical that covered every organ system before making a diagnosis and instituting treatment. Much of this questioning and examining were irrelevant to trauma care and chewed up valuable time that could be better spent averting disaster.

What ATLS taught instead was to treat the greatest threats to life as soon as they were discovered and not to let the lack of a definitive diagnosis delay or prevent the need for an emergency treatment that was obvious.[7]

Styner and his informal group of surgeons, anesthesiologists, orthopedic surgeons, and mobile heart team nurses wrote the chapters that would become the ATLS bible. The course stressed that injury kills in predictable timeframes that dictate the order in which life-threatening emergencies are addressed.

A car wreck victim might present with emergent injuries of the head, chest, and abdomen. The ATLS framework directed the physician to make sure the airway was open first before he moved on to checking for breath sounds on both sides of the chest to detect a life-threatening collapse of the lung. The milieu of an emergency room might be chaotic and distracting, but as long as a physician stayed focused on the steps, he would hopefully catch any potentially fatal threat before it claimed the life of a patient.

A prototype of the course went live in the small town of Auburn, Nebraska (population 3,460), in 1978 and later that year was presented at the University of Nebraska, where it included a skills lab using live animals. Vascular surgeon Dr. Paul Collicott, one of the course's cofounders, took the course to the American College of Surgeons (ACS) Committee on Trauma.[8] The course was then presented to the thirteen regions of the ACS, and within a year the ACS took over and propagated the course across the United States.[9]

Today ATLS is taught to all who are on the front lines of trauma care, including emergency room physicians, surgeons, surgeons-in-training, nurses, and paramedics. Any physician can learn the ATLS method regardless of specialty. More than 1 million physicians in sixty countries (forty thousand physicians per year) have taken the ATLS course, which has become the accepted standard of care for the initial assessment and treatment of the trauma patient worldwide.[10]

One of the side benefits of ATLS is that it provides a common language for those who care for trauma patients so that as patients are transferred from one hospital to another, everyone is on the same page. Styner himself experienced just how meaningful that common language could be when he was on a medical mission in Ayacucho, Peru, in 2003. About a hundred miles from the hospital, two Peruvian marines were wounded when a firefight broke out between the marines and insurgents. Working in a primitive emergency room, Styner and other American physicians who spoke only English worked alongside native Spanish-speaking physicians.

"The common thread was the ATLS language," Styner later said. "It enabled efficient, effective assessment and stabilization . . . so different from our 1976 experience."[11]

WITH MR. X CONTINUING to crater, Dr. Sanchez decided to transfer him to a facility that could provide more experienced trauma care. The nurses started calling around to neighboring hospitals and found one thirty miles away that had a surgeon on standby and could take Mr. X. There was just one problem: How would we get him there alive?

It was 1976. There was no such thing as 9-1-1, and there was no EMS to dispatch. The ambulance that brought Mr. X to the hospital had already been sent to another emergency. The other ambulance services were either too far away or out on calls.

Only one person in town owned a vehicle that could transport Mr. X. Within five minutes the owner of a local funeral home rolled up in a gleaming white-on-white hearse.

WHILE THERE IS SOMETHING unsettling about an undertaker transporting living patients, it was once a common practice in small towns that could not support an independent ambulance service.[12] It was a conundrum that funeral car manufacturers ingeniously capitalized on for most of the twentieth century.

Both hearses and ambulances required rear compartments large enough to accommodate a stretcher or coffin and the accompanying horizontal body. Both required a vehicle with a long wheelbase, extra-wide double doors, and a powerful engine that could haul a heavy load at high speed. Why not design a vehicle that could do both?

The major hearse manufacturers, almost exclusively headquartered in Ohio, used virtually identical bodies for both hearse and ambulance and so were able to streamline production by duplicating the components.[13] In 1964, the Superior Coach Corporation of Lima, Ohio, offered the Pontiac Consort, built on a Pontiac Bonneville chassis, in three configurations—straight ambulance, straight hearse, or a combination hearse/ambulance.

The exterior of combination models could be easily converted by removing the warning lights and sirens from the roof. Interchangeable windows marked "ambulance" could be replaced with solid panels.[14] The interior conversion included the ability to replace a sliding floor plate that created a seat for an attendant with a casket brace.

These early hybrid vehicles, pressed by necessity into dual roles, were rudimentary life-saving chariots by today's standards. What marked them for extinction was not only the increasing sophistication of medical care but also the expansion of the interstate highway system. Throughout the 1950s and '60s the number of highways quadrupled allowing motorists to drive both farther and faster. As a result traffic fatalities started to climb, peaking at approximately fifty thousand per year.

By the 1970s, states began passing legislation requiring new ambulances to be outfitted with expensive equipment, trained personnel, and a dedicated rig built on a van or light truck chassis that could accept the weight of the new standards rather than the hybrids of the past.[15] The 1973 Superior ambulance lineup included the Superior 61, a van conversion created by splitting a Chevy G-30 van down the middle and widening it by fourteen inches.[16]

By 1977 the last of the hearse-style ambulances hit the streets across America. They would soon be replaced with a more utilitarian van-style ambulance. Over the next few years, ambulances evolved in parallel with the EMS system and grew into the large trucks we know today stocked with skilled emergency medical technicians (EMTS) and additional equipment. The funeral car manufacturers of a bygone era returned to the exclusive manufacturing of hearses or, in some cases, diversified into producing armored cars and bulletproof limousines.

NURSE JENKINS RODE in the dark, cavernous cargo compartment with the patient. She was perched on a medical supply bag that she would never be able to get to if she needed anything inside. Besides, she had her hands full bagging Mr. X, steadying the stretcher with her legs, and struggling to palpate a blood pressure.

I was instructed to ride up front to help navigate. The mortician was pushing eighty; he had a hacking cough and a pack of cigarettes to match in his breast pocket. As soon as he backed out of the ambulance bay, he flipped on the deafening siren and immediately steered us into the stream of traffic, passing some cars and dodging others.

About two miles down the road our driver entered the highway access ramp and floored it. As he weaved in and out of traffic, I slid from side to side across the massive front seat, finally bracing myself against the glove compartment. A loud noise like intermittent machine-gun fire emanated from the rear compartment, where the stretcher banged back and forth against the walls.

I wondered how Nurse Jenkins could tell if Mr. X was still alive, much less do anything about it. There were no windows in the back, so it was almost completely dark. Even if she could manage to inflate the blood pressure cuff and palpate the brachial artery, how could she read the numbers on the gauge?

I realized this was not going to be the kind of controlled, efficient ambulance ride I had seen on *Marcus Welby, M.D.*, where fit young men dressed in starched whites with neatly combed hair calmly and competently delivered the patient. This was going to be a race to the finish, a last-ditch attempt to get our patient to the next stop with a heartbeat.

When we neared the city limits of Beaumont, Texas, we slowed down to get our bearings. Nurse Jenkins tapped on the sliding window between our two compartments. She motioned us to hurry up, but we had no GPS, no MapQuest, no iPhone to guide our search. We could rely only on instinct as we cruised up and down the feeder road, looking for a tall red brick building with a cross on top.

Within a few minutes, we found the hospital, and a crowd met us at the emergency ramp and rolled Mr. X away. The three of us walked back to the ambulance, all the adrenaline and emotion of the moment seeping out of us, like bathwater draining from a tub after the plug's been pulled.

After our return, we got the call that told us what we had dreaded all along: Mr. X had died in the operating room shortly after arrival. We had thrown everything we had at him, but it wasn't enough. Mr. X needed to have his chest opened hours earlier by a surgeon who could find the damage, repair it, and deposit him safely in an intensive care unit.

But on that particular day, in a hospital in small-town Texas, that sequence of events could scarcely be imagined, much less achieved.

2 » THE LESSONS OF WAR

ON JULY 21, 1861, the grassy plains of Manassas, Virginia, were transformed from a bucolic landscape into a human slaughterhouse at the Battle of Bull Run, the first major battle of the Civil War. Wounded soldiers were left bleeding, moaning in pain and dying on the battlefield for days and weeks without the benefit of the most basic medical attention.[1] What made the gruesome scenario particularly chilling was the unfolding realization that no one was coming back to rescue them. By battle's end the designated rescue vehicles, repurposed horse-drawn wagons, were nowhere in sight.

If the wounded were going to get off the battlefield, they would have to drag themselves over twenty-seven miles of what was now enemy-occupied territory, without food, water, or so much as an aspirin. Incredibly, hundreds managed to do so, all the way to Washington, D.C., enough to horrify citizens of our nation's capital who watched out their windows as soldiers staggered through the streets in torn and bloodied uniforms. In the aftermath of one of the worst battles of the war, the phrase "walking wounded" entered the American lexicon and stayed.

EVERY WAR IS A trauma lesson. Along with devastating injuries comes an opportunity to improve the care of the wounded. But first the hurdles that come with taking care of troops on the battlefield must be negotiated—training a competent medical corps, constructing hospitals, and figuring out the logistics of evacuating the wounded. Each new combat setting poses unfamiliar challenges that offer both a proving ground and a laboratory for military physicians. The cost of lessons learned is steep, measured in lives and limbs, as the tedious work of grappling with never-before-seen injuries begins and drags on until a remedy is found. But physicians are innovators, and war inspires them to invent solutions that, in the long run, benefit all of society.

World War I brought us the underpinnings of plastic surgery. World War II inspired the wholesale production of penicillin and the creation of a national blood bank. The Vietnam War brought the recognition of shock lung and the first widespread repair of extremity blood vessels. And the wars in Iraq and Afghanistan delivered advanced forward surgical care and a new generation of prostheses that can move with the strength and precision of real extremities.

THERE IS NO better example of the human costs of war than the Civil War, a conflict that overwhelmed the medical profession with trauma and disease on a mass scale and challenged it to respond. An estimated 750,000 soldiers died during the war —one-third due to injuries and two-thirds as a result of disease. The medical department of the U.S. Army could hardly be held responsible for the flood of casualties that broke through the levees of its expertise and capacity.

At the outset there were only a hundred physicians in the U.S. Army Medical Corps, and a third of them resigned to join the Confederate army.[2] Those left behind had virtually no operative experience, and most had never seen a bullet wound.

During the first major battle of the war, the Battle of Bull Run, Dr. William S. King, medical director for the Army of the Potomac, watched in disbelief as wounded bodies began to pile up.

Expecting only a brief skirmish in what many thought would be a rout of the Confederate army, he had failed to draft evacuation plans, set up postbattle aid stations, or designate field hospitals. How was he going to catch up now?

King's only choice was to scramble. He dispatched soldiers to commandeer Sudley Church, only a few miles away. They removed pews, gathered hay from nearby fields to serve as bedding, and brought in water. Within hours this improvised field hospital was overflowing with wounded men and three other buildings had to be converted. An untrained medical staff worked with no medications and few supplies.

As night fell, the Confederate army advanced on Sudley Church and volunteers were told to evacuate to Washington. Only a handful of surgeons remained behind to care for hundreds of wounded.[3] One of those who stayed was William Williams Keen, a twenty-four-year-old medical student from Jefferson Medical College (now Thomas Jefferson School of Medicine) who only two weeks before had been sworn in to the Army Medical Department at the level of assistant surgeon.[4] When Keen, who, by his own admission, was "as green as the grass around me," arrived at the church, he found in front of the pulpit an operating table hastily constructed of two boards straddling boxes on either end. A gallery of injured men looked down on the surgeons as they worked. Women from the neighborhood nursed the wounded. Keen immediately jumped in to assist in a shoulder joint amputation, putting pressure on the axillary artery when it started spurting as the cut was made.

Later he was bandaging an arm fractured by a bullet when suddenly a herd of soldiers came running down the road shouting, "The rebs are after us." Keen's patient wrenched his arm away and took off at a dead run, his bandage unwinding as he fled.[5]

THE ARMY MEDICAL DEPARTMENT mirrored the state of American medicine in the 1860s. Medical education and training was primitive. There were no national standards for the training of physicians, and numerous factions of practitioners, such as allopaths (the mainstream practitioners of today), homeopaths, hydropaths, and herbalists, competed with each other.[6] Due to religious taboos and superstition, cadavers for dissection were scarce, leaving physicians with little knowledge of anatomy. The idea that the country could muster a force to competently deal with trauma victims was a distant dream.

With the advent of the Civil War, physicians from private practices in small towns and cities volunteered to fill the gaps of the military medical force, but few had any practical experience in trauma or epidemics. As the war progressed, medical students and trainees with even less experience were pressed into service.

This was our first generation of trauma surgeons. Like modern-day interns on their first night of ER call in a busy intercity hospital, they were not prepared for the human wreckage rolling through the doors. Many had never held a scalpel or tied a ligature. There was no equipment, little in the way of supplies, and no coordinated plan of action.

Surgeons had to carry their own tools in hinged wooden boxes lined with felt like those made to nuzzle the family silver. But instead of cutlery appointed with scrolled flowers, these boxes held knives with foot-long blades, bone-grasping rongeur clamps, and hacksaws, files, and rasps to smooth the rough surface of a naked stalk of protruding bone.

EVERY WAR HAS its surprises, the unforeseen events that emerge out of a change of circumstances and lead to unanticipated misery—a weapons upgrade that produces a new pattern of injury, a shift in enemy tactics that seems impossible to defend against, a contagious disease that ravages close-quartered camps, a blast of weather that freezes bodies into lifeless bricks.

In World War I, trench warfare led to epidemics of disease and to horrendous head and neck wounds caused by unprotected soldiers peering over a trench. Vietnam brought "bouncing Bettys," underground grenades that lopped off feet and legs. Iraq introduced us to improvised explosive devices (IEDS), remote-controlled bombs that blew off every part of a soldier that wasn't armored and rattled his brains.

One of the biggest surprises of the Civil War was the staggering number of wounded that piled up after every major battle—ten thousand casualties during the first four hours of the Battle of Antietam, a number more in keeping with a natural disaster than a military firefight.[7] Even the most organized and efficient of medical teams would have had difficulty sorting through that many dead and wounded. The toxic combination of game-changing weaponry and stalled military tactics had set the stage for unexpected casualties.

For the previous one hundred years, wars had been fought with the musket, a cumbersome single-shot weapon that could not be fired until a concoction of gunpowder, paper, and bullet had been shoved down the barrel and a fresh firing cap placed near the trigger. The musket was accurate to a distance of only fifty yards and kicked out a round ball that traveled like a bad knuckleball, zig-zagging in flight with only a prayer of reaching the target.

But in 1861, along came the new Springfield .58-caliber rifle, potentially much deadlier and more accurate thanks to the introduction of the minié ball, a half-inch, unjacketed lead bullet outfitted with an expanding skirt that allowed a tight fit with the barrel. On firing, the ball would spin, increasing its velocity to up to 950 feet per second. Overnight, the rifle's accuracy increased to six hundred yards, the length of six football fields.[8]

Both Union and Confederate forces had the upgraded rifles, but they continued to fight in the same shoulder-to-shoulder formations—soldiers lined up three rows deep to allow for reloading. The new high-powered rifles easily picked off men in such close groupings.

Minié balls did not punch neatly through the skin like a bullet striking a paper target at a gun range. They flattened out and made fist-sized holes on impact, ripping apart skin and subcutaneous tissue, transecting nerves and blood vessels and splintering bones. Very little was known about how to realign, cast, or splint a broken bone, much less how to repair transected blood vessels or perform a skin graft or any other reconstructive procedure. The overall effect was a mangled mess of a wound that outstripped any known method of repair.

In an era that predated antiseptic techniques, severely damaged limbs posed the danger of life-threatening infection. So surgeons defaulted to the only life-saving operation they knew and had the tools to perform—limb amputation.

Twelve percent of all injured soldiers underwent amputations; by comparison, in World War I only 1.7 percent of those wounded lost a limb.[9] Of the 174,200 gunshot wounds to the extremities in Union soldiers, almost 30,000 required amputation.[10]

Amputations were carried out under primitive conditions on makeshift operating tables in a large room of a house, in a barn, or in a tent.[11] For lack of space and light they might even be performed outdoors, where crowds often gathered. Men stood in line for the procedure and watched as fellow soldiers' limbs piled up nearby, a gruesome reminder of the toll of war.

Union General Ulysses S. Grant himself had trouble taking in the grisly sights of a battlefield hospital he visited on the eve of the Battle of Shiloh: "All night wounded men were being brought in, their wounds dressed, a leg or an arm amputated as the case might require, and everything being done to save life or alleviate suffering. The sight was more unendurable than encountering the enemy's fire, and I returned to my tree in the rain."[12]

Once a soldier gave his consent to the operation, he was hastily held down by several men until it was finished. Later in the war, patients were anesthetized with ether or chloroform dripped on a cloth and held over their nose. Even then speed in execution was essential because the patient might wake up and start moving midprocedure. Experienced surgeons could complete the operation in three minutes.

THE LACK OF PREPARATION for the wounded at Bull Run outraged the United States Sanitary Commission, a humanitarian organization that provided supplies and acted as a watchdog for the health and hygiene of the military. Sanitary Commission members became increasingly vocal in their criticism and lobbied Congress to do something about the emerging pattern of neglected wounded.

Enter newly appointed Surgeon General William Hammond, who took office on April 28, 1862, nine months after the First Battle of Bull Run. Hammond, having served as the chair of anatomy and physiology at the University of Maryland, had an academic as well as a military background.[13] Forceful, direct, and efficient, he was a cutting-edge, science-oriented change-agent, a man hellbent on reforming the army medical department.

Hammond enacted a wholesale upgrade to what had been an uneven physician workforce by subjecting all new applicants to a multipart entrance examination. No longer would he be accepting just anyone who wandered in the door with MD behind his name.

Early in his tenure, he saw the potential to compile a treasure trove of medical data unequaled in the history of American medicine. On May 21, 1862, he issued a directive establishing the Army Medical Museum and ordering medical officers to collect and forward to the office of the Surgeon General "all specimens of morbid anatomy, surgical or medical . . . together with projectiles and foreign bodies removed."[14]

Hammond also required medical officers to submit case reports, autopsies, and other descriptions along with the specimens. These written descriptions and the data derived from them would be published in what was, in effect, our nation's first trauma textbook.[15] The final product, *The Medical and Surgical History of the*

War of the Rebellion (1861–1865), a six-volume, 4,883-page work, weighed a total of fifty-five pounds and exceeded in size and scope anything Hammond could have imagined.[16]

One of Hammond's best moves was tapping his former classmate Jonathan Letterman to be medical director of the Army of the Potomac. Like most physicians, Letterman had virtually no wartime experience, and the only wounds he had treated before the Civil War were from arrows launched by Apaches in what is now New Mexico. With his appointment came the instant responsibility for the medical care of fifty thousand soldiers.

On July 1, 1862, Letterman arrived at Harrison's Landing and walked in on a disaster of a medical department. General Robert E. Lee had just routed the Army of the Potomac at the Seven Days' Battle, just east of Richmond, Virginia. There were thirteen thousand casualties from the campaign, and thousands of wounded soldiers had been laid out along the James River.

His first week on the job he ordered a thousand tents and two hundred ambulances. He evacuated the wounded to offshore steamships that served as hospitals. To combat scurvy and build up the weakened troops, he mandated that trained cooks prepare nutritious meals that included fresh fruits and vegetables.

Letterman organized the first trained ambulance corps, taking control from individual regiments and placing the corps under a central authority so that training could be standardized. Two trained attendants and a driver manned each ambulance. Neither the ambulance nor the personnel could be conscripted to other duties.

A medical system that met the needs of the Army of the Potomac was finally starting to take shape, but before it could be fully realized, commanding officer General George McClellan was ordered back to Washington and what remained of his army was assigned to join the Army of Virginia. Letterman, now a medical director in name only, was left hanging as another major battle, the Second Battle of Bull Run, loomed.

THE SECOND BATTLE of Bull Run proved to be even costlier than the first, leaving ten thousand soldiers dead, wounded, or captive. In the aftermath of yet another military disaster, Lincoln reinstated McClellan, and Letterman resumed his role as medical director. His next insurmountable challenge was to reassemble his fledgling medical system, in time for the Battle of Antietam, only two weeks away.

In the days before the battle, Letterman surveyed Antietam Creek and the nearby battlefield. He projected where the greatest numbers of soldiers would be wounded and planned evacuation routes to get them off the battlefield quickly. He scouted churches, farmhouses, barns, and public buildings and organized them into a network of almost a hundred hospitals and aid stations. He assigned personnel and surgeons to each location and had supplies delivered.[17]

Under Letterman's plan the ambulance corps would pick up the wounded and take them to the nearest regimental aid station, where surgeons would control bleeding and clean and dress their wounds. From there, ambulances would take them to field hospitals within a couple of miles of the battlefield, where wounds were further cleaned and amputations performed. Hospital trains and ships would transport the wounded from the field hospitals to the hospitals located in the rear in major cities.

The fighting began at 5 a.m. on September 17, 1862. By 9 a.m. there were ten thousand Union casualties. Letterman's assistant rode from one field hospital to the next and sent reports back to Letterman about the location of the wounded. Letterman directed ambulances to retrieve injured soldiers from the front aid stations and hospitals that were overflowing with patients and deliver them to the larger hospitals in the rear. By the time the sun set on what was later referred to as "America's bloodiest day," more than twenty-three thousand Union and Confederate soldiers had been injured or killed.[18]

The next day there were still hundreds of wounded soldiers on the battlefield, but every bed in Letterman's hospitals was full. There had also been glitches, like the failure to get boxcar-loads of medical supplies because a railroad bridge had been destroyed.

And Letterman was forced to commandeer private homes to house even more wounded because many were too unstable to be transported over long distances by wagons, trains, and ships as planned. But in less than two days, the ambulance corps evacuated 8,350 wounded Union soldiers and 2,000 Confederates from the field and, by twenty-four hours after the battle, the entire battlefield was cleared of wounded.

Letterman's system had been strained to capacity, but it had expanded when necessary and responded to the increased flow of casualties, and in the end it was judged a resounding success. This success would be repeated in December 1862 at Fredericksburg, where the wounded were evacuated within twelve hours. It was repeated at Gettysburg, where nearly twenty-one thousand wounded Union soldiers and Confederate prisoners were evacuated and treated.

The Civil War's toll in suffering and death is unmatched in our nation's history, but the conflict shined a much-needed spotlight on the care of the wounded, exposed its weaknesses, and jump-started the modern era of American medicine. Perhaps the most important lesson of war was the one learned from Letterman and passed on to the armies of the future. Preparing for war didn't just mean enlisting soldiers, acquiring arms, and planning an attack strategy. Preparing for war also meant having a plan to rescue the wounded and preparing facilities to care for them. Letterman had installed the first rudimentary trauma system, and for decades into the future his system would continue to transform the care of the wounded.

3 » THE WEAKEST LINK

"1 A.M., PATIENT'S blood pressure has dropped to 70/40; I have called the doctor again."

The nurse knew her patient was in trouble, but she couldn't even start a blood transfusion without an order. And there was no one else to call. All she could do was wait, and by the time the surgeon arrived an hour later her patient had died.[1]

Epidemiologist Sue Baker was reviewing the medical chart of the forty-year-old male car crash victim when she came across the entry written by an emergency room nurse at a rural Maryland hospital. Moments later she watched as the medical examiner drew his scalpel across the victim's abdomen. As soon as he had penetrated the layers of muscle, blood started to well up and out of the incision. The pathologist reached inside with his gloved hand, felt around, and found the ragged edges of the culprit organ. The patient had bled out from a ruptured spleen, an injury he might have survived if he had gotten to the operating room in time.

The year was 1972. Baker was working in the Baltimore medical examiner's office, where she watched autopsies in the morning and pored over logbooks in the afternoon, looking for clues. *Why were so many people dying on America's roads? What were the injuries that were killing them? And what could be done to change these bleak outcomes?*

In an era where trauma care was still haphazard and unde-fined, ambulances dropped trauma patients at the nearest hos-pital regardless of how ill-equipped it might be to care for them. Baker had seen avoidable deaths like this one way too many times and was sniffing out a pattern. Suspecting there were more cases buried in the logbooks, she put together a research team—herself, two trauma surgeons, and a medical examiner. She did the initial digging and came up with a list of thirty-three fatalities from isolated abdominal injuries sustained in car crashes. The physicians classified the injuries as potentially survivable or not, and when the team analyzed the data, Baker's hunch was con-firmed: Half of those who had died might have been saved with timely treatment.

She published her findings, including the fact that the larger metropolitan hospitals with in-house trauma surgeons rarely reported survivable abdominal injuries that resulted in death. Those injuries came from small, understaffed community hospi-tals like the one where the Maryland nurse had tried in vain to get a doctor to respond. Baker and her team concluded that patients with major injuries such as victims of car crashes should be taken to larger hospitals that were best equipped to treat them.[2]

To understand Sue Baker you have to wind the tape back to 1967. Sue Baker—wife, mother of three, and a grad student in public health at Johns Hopkins—tagged along with her husband on a trip to Annapolis, Maryland. Professor Tim Baker, an inter-national health expert, was testifying at a legislative hearing in support of a bill that would allow police to test motorists for al-cohol consumption. It was during those hearings that Baker first heard the alarming statistic: Fifty thousand people a year were dying in car crashes.

"I was horrified and I realized that Hopkins wasn't doing any-thing about it—no research in injury prevention, no courses, not even a single lecture."[3]

Public health initiatives in the 1960s were targeting diseases, particularly communicable diseases like smallpox. The concept that injuries could be analyzed and the root causes attacked, just as with diseases, was virtually nonexistent. Injury prevention was an orphan area of study in public health, the perfect playground for a young woman who was raised to "figure out how things worked" in her father's workshop.

When she graduated with a master's of public health from Johns Hopkins in 1968, Baker headed to the City of Baltimore morgue, a logical place to start to unravel how injuries were killing people. If she could find out the causes and circumstances, perhaps solutions could be found. She spent the next twelve years digging through records and looking at broken bodies. It was a journey that took her to places she never dreamed she'd find herself in.[4]

Like much that Baker researched and wrote about for the next five decades, the paper on avoidable trauma deaths provided trailblazing information that, in the right hands, would impact the treatment of injury victims. Dr. R Adams Cowley, the first head of the Maryland Shock Trauma Unit, seized on Baker's article and used it to persuade government officials to implement the first statewide trauma system in 1970, one that would direct the most severely injured from the streets to his trauma unit.[5] The innovative program saved hundreds of thousands of lives and became a model for regionalized trauma care.

Baker wasn't an MD and didn't work in a medical school, but her unembellished words printed in the pages of medical journals drew attention to injury and shook up the way people thought about them. Over time she deduced that what led to most "accidents" was actually a chain of events proceeding toward a predictable outcome. If the chain could be interrupted, perhaps injury could be averted altogether.

She paid attention to specific details that would lead her to the weakest link in the chain. If the data showed, for example, that there had been a large number of motor vehicle fatalities at the same spot on a street, Baker would get in her car, drive over, and see what was going on. She might discover something that others had missed, like a curve on a downhill slope that headed straight into a tree. Installing a simple guardrail on the road in front of the tree could disrupt the pattern. And that would become Baker's trademark—studying the data, uncovering the weakest links in our daily lives, and setting up guardrails in front of them.

THE WORD "TRAUMA" conjures up heart-thumping scenes complete with ambulances, emergency rooms, surgeons, and life-saving operations, but in the shadows is a parallel field made up of injury scientists who pursue the goal of making our world safer. These epidemiologists, engineers, physicians, consumer advocates, and lawmakers have spent their careers chipping away at the causes and conditions that lead to needless death and suffering and coming up with ways to prevent injury from occurring in the first place.

Engineer Hugh DeHaven's view of injury and how to prevent it depended not only on his training as an engineer but also on his personal experiences with trauma. In 1917, when he was training as a volunteer pilot with the Canadian Flying Corps, his plane collided with another, and both crashed. The other pilot was killed, but DeHaven survived with two broken legs and extensive intra-abdominal injuries.[6]

While he was hospitalized for six months recovering from liver, pancreas, and gallbladder injuries, he reflected on the fact that the safety belt he had been wearing had an oversized pointed buckle that had penetrated his abdomen on impact and skewered his organs. He began to daydream about redesigning the cabin of a plane to minimize injuries.

When he left the service, DeHaven became an inventor specializing in packaging design and developed a device that could bind wooden shipping crates with wire to hold them together during transport. He decided to apply his expertise to vehicle safety when he witnessed a rollover car crash in 1953. The driver's head was slammed into a protruding steel knob on the dashboard, leaving a wide gash in his forehead.

"People know more about protecting eggs in transit than they do about protecting human heads," he observed.[7] He believed that if humans were "packaged" better within a vehicle, their chances of being injured would decrease. Why not apply to automobile passengers the same engineering principles used to safeguard cargo?

DeHaven tested his theory by dropping eggs from ceiling height in his kitchen onto a half-inch-thick piece of foam. None of the eggs broke. He then reenacted the experiment on a larger scale, dropping eggs from a building at a height of one hundred feet onto a three-inch-deep rubber mat. Again, the eggs landed intact, demonstrating that with even a modest amount of cushioning, a fragile object could withstand impact.[8]

DeHaven collected data about survivors of falls from heights in an attempt to understand what had kept them alive. If he spotted an article in the newspaper about someone surviving after jumping or falling from a window, he would visit the accident scene himself, inspect it for clues and, if possible, visit the person in the hospital.[9]

In 1942, he published a report of eight cases in which seven victims survived falls from heights of 50 to 150 feet.[10] He discovered that it wasn't the height of the fall that determined the extent of injury but, rather, the surface they hit. Five of the victims jumped, and two fell accidentally, but in almost every case the impact was cushioned because the victim either struck an intervening object such as a car, a box, or a fence or (in two cases) landed in soft dirt. A forty-two-year-old woman who jumped from the sixth floor landed in a garden on her side, indenting the ground four inches. After the fall, the woman, sat up in dismay and said, "Six stories and not hurt."[11]

DeHaven's study documented that humans could survive

great impacts and that survival wasn't just a matter of luck.[12] To minimize injury, the force of impact must be uniformly distributed and reduced by the ambient environment.

In the 1950s DeHaven used package design principles to propose optimal features of a crashworthy vehicle.[13] Just as a package should stay closed to prevent spilling its contents during transport, so should a car door stay shut. This meant having stronger doors and better locks to prevent passenger ejection. The same way the inside of a package is cushioned to absorb jostling, so must the interior of a car be padded where a passenger is liable to slam into the surface during a crash. This translated into padded dashboards and recessed control knobs. The same way items were held in place when a container fell in transit, a passenger must be restrained to keep from being thrown around inside the vehicle on impact.

DeHaven put his principles of crash survival into action when he worked with Roger Griswold in 1951 to invent the first three-point shoulder and lap safety belt. Volvo further developed the three-point safety belt and made it standard equipment on all models by 1959.[14]

Because of resistance from industry, most of DeHaven's visionary ideas were not implemented in his lifetime, but he pioneered a new field of engineering—crash-survival design—that would ultimately make cars and planes safer in the event of an accident.[15] More importantly, he served as an important role model for the next generation of injury prevention enthusiasts, including an up-and-coming epidemiologist named Sue Baker.

EARLY ON, IN 1971, Baker was collecting data on fatally injured drivers and noticed that the last four victims she'd reviewed all had tattoos.[16] She hadn't meant to study them, but there they were, flashing before her eyes and begging to be noticed. So she went back over her data and recoded all her subjects for the presence of tattoos, and that's when the pattern appeared: Tattooed drivers who were fatally injured were more likely than nontattooed drivers to be at fault in car crashes.

She wrote up a grant proposal to study driver responsibility and sent it to Dr. William Haddon, a medical doctor and engineer who was approaching traffic safety from a different angle. In 1966, Haddon was the director of the New York State Health Department when he was tapped by President Lyndon Johnson to lead the newly created National Highway Traffic Safety Administration. He was responsible for instituting the first federal crash safety standards and eventually headed up the Insurance Institute for Highway Safety.

Haddon eschewed terms such as "luck" or "accident" to describe injury and focused on causative factors with an eye toward prevention. Modern-day medicine methodically attacked disease at the level of causation—for example, preventing the spread of the poliomyelitis virus that caused polio. But for some reason the medical community resisted doing the same with injury so that it too could be controlled at the source. Haddon would change that paradigm.

In 1968, Haddon derived his now classic matrix to analyze and mitigate causative factors in the preinjury, injury, and postinjury phases.[17] Precrash analysis for car wrecks might entail improving driving conditions to prevent accidents in the first place, such as safer tires, better lighting, banked curves on highways, and reflectors on guardrails. Factors that affected the crash phase included air bags, seatbelts, and padded dashboards—anything that protected a passenger during impact. The third, postcrash phase concerned maximizing salvage of the injured passenger— for example, the availability of emergency medical care that provided prompt resuscitation and transportation to a trauma center.

As Haddon's philosophy spread, so did the proliferation of injury prevention experts, who began to adopt a more rational and analytical approach to controlling injuries. Students of public health embraced Haddon's matrix and expanded its use beyond injury dynamics and into a host of other public health threats, including infectious disease and violent crime.

When Haddon received Sue Baker's letter asking for ten thousand dollars to fund her study on tattoos, alcohol, and driver responsibility for crashes, he recognized the project's potential and instructed his deputy Bob Brenner to call her two days later.

"Dr. Haddon wants to fund this. Just send us a budget," he said to her.[18]

And thus began a seventeen-year alliance between two of the most brilliant minds in the history of injury prevention and public safety. The collaboration was brought to a premature end in 1985 by Haddon's untimely death from kidney failure at age fifty-eight, but Baker continued on for another thirty years.[19]

JOHN PAUL STAPP picked up where Hugh DeHaven left off when he became a human crash test dummy riding in the seat of the rocket-propelled sled *Sonic Wind No. 1* in 1954. The ride took less than seven seconds from start to finish, but screaming down a track at a blazing 632 miles per hour and being slammed to a complete standstill stunned the pilot. The sudden deceleration had yanked Stapp's body with a measured force of 43G, the equivalent of smashing into a brick wall at 70 miles per hour. While flashbulbs went off in all directions on the test track at Holloman Air Force Base in the New Mexico desert, Stapp was lifted from the crash sled, placed on a stretcher, loaded into an ambulance, and driven to a nearby medical facility.[20]

Stapp was not a daredevil in pursuit of a Guinness world record, even though this extraordinary feat earned him the title "The Fastest Man on Earth," the cover of *Time* magazine, and numerous accolades for bravery. This air force colonel, medical doctor, and PhD biophysicist, was, in fact, a pioneering researcher in the limits of human injury tolerance, trying to determine the maximum speed at which a pilot could safely eject from an airplane while also testing the efficacy of shoulder harnesses.

Stapp's experiments placed him in a great deal of danger. When a fast-moving body comes to an abrupt stop, as in a head-on collision, internal organs continue to move forward and can actually tear or stretch away from their roots.[21] Severe deceleration injuries can cause the aorta, the largest blood vessel in the body, to rupture and the blood vessels of the brain to shear. Intra-abdominal organs including the spleen, kidney, and small intestine can also be torn in a sudden deceleration.

A video of Stapp's postride physical shows a doughy, middle-aged male, his round face sporting two black eyes, smiling and answering questions while a physician documents the damage. His body was covered with blisters from where dirt had penetrated his wool flak suit and lodged under his skin. The whites of his eyes had hemorrhaged, a so-called red-out, when his eyeballs pitched forward in their sockets and then snapped back into place.

"It felt as though my eyes were being pulled out of my head, about the same sort of sensation as when a molar is yanked," Stapp said later.[22] Doctors feared that Stapp would be permanently blinded, but his vision started to return within a few hours.

As Stapp pointed out, the human body is made up of a wide variety of tissues with complex architecture.[23] Because of human beings' unique composition, Stapp, like many other researchers, believed that there was no substitute for human volunteers in testing the limits of human endurance. Human volunteers were especially valuable for determining injury thresholds and setting limits on how much force a human could stand before being injured.

Human volunteer testing was widespread during the 1950s. In other human trials, subjects were strapped to a vibrating "shake table" while sequential X-rays were taken to measure the deformation of organs within the chest and abdominal cavities.[24] Others lying supine withstood the impact of a weighted vest dropped from a height of three feet onto their torsos so that mechanical waves cresting through the chest and abdomen could be measured.[25]

Everyone knew that the *Sonic Wind No. 1* was only one equipment malfunction—a torn harness strap, a cracked helmet, or a derailment—away from delivering its passenger to the graveyard. By at least one account some sled riders had sustained injuries so severe they had ended up in shock or disabled.[26] But Stapp, the son of two Baptist missionaries, was imbued with a spirit of self-sacrifice for the greater good. He infused his research with the same fervor that had been displayed by his parents in the mountains of Brazil, where they taught at the American Baptist College.

Over the course of twenty-nine high-speed rides, Stapp broke ribs, suffered concussions, lost six fillings, developed an abdominal wall hernia, fractured his tailbone, shattered a wrist (twice), and undoubtedly sustained other occult injuries that were underdiagnosed without today's sophisticated diagnostic tools.

In 1955, the year after his record-breaking ride, he started the Stapp Car Crash Conference to share his data and ideas with biomechanical engineers, automotive manufacturers, traffic and safety councils, and physicians and other trauma experts.[27] The fifty-eighth annual Stapp conference was held in 2014, and it continues today as a forum for the discussion of the causes and mechanisms of injury.[28]

AS BAKER'S CAREER steadily marched along, she uncovered information about carbon monoxide poisoning associated with the rusted-out bottoms of cars, childhood asphyxiation from choking on hot dogs, the dangers of accidental overdoses from easily accessed pill bottles, house fires, and risk factors for dying at the wheel while driving. Along the way she became a professor of public health and in 1987 founded the Center for Injury Research and Policy at the Johns Hopkins School of Public Health. The media would inevitably publicize her findings and provoke a flurry of attention that would bring about change. Among her 250 papers, several stood out as game changers in the world of trauma.

In 1970, while still at the office of the medical examiner, Baker began a large-scale study of traffic deaths in Baltimore, not really knowing where it would lead. She compared the death rates of patients who had sustained more than one major injury with those who had only one and found that having even one additional injury significantly increased the chances of dying, even if neither injury was, by itself, considered fatal.

She was able to develop a formula to calculate an injury severity score based on a patient's injuries so that trauma surgeons could compare the mortality of similar groups of patients and evaluate methods of resuscitation and definitive care. Her paper "The Injury Severity Score: A Method for Describing Patients with Multiple Injuries and Evaluating Emergency Care," published in 1974, has been the most frequently cited article from the *Journal of Trauma* since its inception.[29] For someone who more than once was mistaken for the wife of a trauma surgeon, rather than a presenter, at national trauma meetings, she made up considerable ground.

Baker's other game-changing paper came out of what she discovered about children who died in car crashes. She had reviewed case after case of infant fatalities where mothers cradled babies in their laps with the intention of keeping them safe. But in a head-on crash, the baby became a human airbag, absorbing the impact before it could reach the mother. Baker was the first to document that the death rate for motor vehicle occupants age zero to twelve was highest for children less than six months old (9 in every 100,000) and gradually dropped with increasing age to 3 in every 100,000.

In 1979, at the time her paper "Motor Vehicle Occupant Deaths in Young Children" was published in the journal *Pediatrics*, only one state, Tennessee, had passed a child restraint law (1978). Baker's data exposed a national tragedy that required urgent action.

What followed was a decade of engineering, legislative, and medical attention to the problem. In 1981 the American Academy of Pediatrics began its "First Ride, Safe Ride" program to promote the use of infant car seats for the initial discharge from the hospital after birth, and by 1985 every state had passed some version of a child passenger safety law.[30] There was still much work to be done in terms of both car seat design and position and the effectiveness of legislation, but it was a promising start.

BAKER'S *INJURY FACT BOOK*, published in 1984, was the first resource to report trauma fatalities due to all mechanisms in the fifty states. Not only was the book a stark wakeup call, documenting the magnitude of the injury threat to public safety; it also served as a valuable reference tool. Baker prepared maps depicting the concentration of particular injuries in the United States by location. If a legislator wanted to compare the death rate in a particular state from firearm homicides to nonfirearm homicides, he could simply put the two maps side by side.

One such map pinpointed where small planes had crashed across the country. Baker was surprised to find that between 1964 and 1987, 232 small planes had crashed within fifty miles of Aspen, Colorado.[31] Further digging revealed that while commercial and military plane crashes were extensively investigated, there was very little known about the crashes of privately owned planes. Baker's investigative instincts started to engage. The only problem was that she knew nothing about flying planes. In her mind it would be next to impossible to become an expert in aviation safety without a pilot's license, so in typical Baker fashion, at age fifty-six, she began flying lessons at Baltimore Washington International Airport.

Halfway through her lessons she was involved in two mishaps while at the controls, both due to mechanical malfunctions. Baker was shaken, and she grounded herself after the second near crash. It was her husband, Tim, who gently nudged her to finish the training, telling her she wouldn't be satisfied until she had a pilot's license in hand. She then collaborated with pilot Margaret Lamb, an expert in mountain flying. The two flew Lamb's plane over crash sites and through mountain passes and interviewed pilots and instructors at small airports in Colorado.

They discovered two key pieces of data. First, many pilots failed to use shoulder harnesses in addition to lap belts, which led to a 37 percent increase in the probability of being killed in a crash. Second, many pilots didn't understand how high altitude and warm weather affected a plane's ability to climb over rising terrain. They routinely overloaded their low-powered four-seater aircrafts, thus leading to avoidable crashes.[32]

Baker called for better surveillance of civil aviation crashes so that mechanical factors could be identified and preventive measures instituted and recommended restraint systems to prevent head-injury related fatalities, increased training for pilots of sightseeing helicopters, planes, and hot-air balloons, and more stringent regulations for commuter aircraft.

FOR THOSE WHO WONDER if Baker's and her colleagues' efforts have been successful, consider the following: In the past fifty years, the highway death rate has dropped by 80 percent. The motor vehicle death rate in infants less than a year of age dropped by 40 percent in less than three decades. The number of deaths from aspirin toxicity in victims less than five years old dropped from 144 in 1960 to zero in 2010.[33]

As impressive as it is to reflect on how Baker's own research has made the world safer, the ripple effect of her work is equally remarkable. Throughout her career, she has mentored hundreds of individuals and instilled her own brand of injury prevention focus and drive.

Dr. Flaura Winston is one example. She is a pediatrician and a biomedical engineer who, early in her career, asked Baker to "help me put these two careers together." Winston went on to apply both areas of expertise to preventing childhood injuries from car crashes and was the first to recognize the danger of airbags to children in forward-facing seats. Now a professor of pediatrics at the Children's Hospital of Philadelphia and the director of the Center for Child Injury Prevention Studies for the National Science Foundation, she has brought attention to distracted driving in teenagers, the optimal positioning and restraints for infants and children in cars, the vulnerabilities of novice drivers, and post-traumatic stress disorder (PTSD) in children and their parents after injury.[34]

Epidemiologist Dr. Janine Jagger, another Baker mentee, was one of the first to document the risk of needlestick injuries to healthcare workers in the 1980s. She developed a surveillance system to track needlestick injuries and bloodborne exposures and contributed to the invention of the first generation of safe hypodermic needles.[35] She was awarded a MacArthur fellowship in 2002 in recognition of her pioneering work in healthcare worker safety.

Dr. Carol Runyan, director of the University of North Carolina Injury Prevention Research Center for twenty-two years, first studied under Baker as a graduate student in public health, where she researched burn injuries in teenaged workers.[36] She became a leading scholar in violence as a public health threat, particularly on college campuses.

There is a common theme that runs through the Baker family tree of public health researchers. Whether the research subjects are healthcare workers, automobile passengers, or victims of violence, preventing injury does not depend on changing human behavior. Baker passed on her core philosophy: It's not who you can blame but what you can change. Preventing injuries is about changing the environment, not people.

At eighty-five, Baker continues to be an active scholar and to take on mentees. Most recently, Commander Jennifer Proctor of the U.S. Public Health Service met with her about how to make national parks safer. National park officials have been cautioning park visitors for decades about potential hazards in the wild with posted warnings, letters, emails, and reminders from park rangers. But visitors still climb over barriers and fall to their deaths, fail to carry enough water and succumb to heatstroke, or slip into rushing waters and drown. Adhering to her philosophy, Baker advised the young engineer not to waste her time battling human nature; rather, she should look at ways to provide safety nets for the misguided decisions tourists will make that will inevitably get them into trouble.

4 » LEARNING TO FLY

FAR OUT PAST the lights of Houston, we reach a stretch of woods thick with pine and the damp chill of night. We circle the area until a small dot of light appears—the accident scene, lit only by EMS headlights and the crimson glow of flares. As the pilot threads the Twin Star through a gap in the trees, the silhouette of an overturned pickup truck comes into view. With the rotors still thumping, I grab my bag and jump into a swirl of dirt and rocks, looking for a stretcher, a body, a patient to rescue.

"He was out riding around with his girlfriend when the truck flipped," an EMT reports. "She ran several miles to get help. We haven't been able to get him out yet, but he's not looking too good in there."

I crouch down a couple of feet away and look into the cab of the overturned pickup, gasoline fumes wafting out of the soaked seats. I crawl toward the wreckage through the scatter of glass and metal, picking my way through the debris.

"Wait a minute, Doc. We're not sure this thing is going to stay up," he says, referring to the truck balanced awkwardly in the middle of the dirt road.

"I can't check him out from here," I tell him. "I've got to get closer."

I look inside the car window and find a young man in his late teens slouched behind the steering wheel. His long dark hair is parted down the middle, his face smooth and pale except for a jagged laceration where his forehead smacked the windshield. An unopened can of Budweiser juts out of the breast pocket of his fatigue jacket.

He doesn't move or open his eyes except for an occasional labored breath. I move farther in and place two fingers on his neck and find a faint pulse. Both pupils are dilated and nonreactive. I pry his mouth open and see a pool of blood sloshing back and forth in the back of his throat. Instead of vocal cords there are only tattered remnants, floating. At the very least he has a severe head injury and maybe a broken neck. If we can start CPR, open an airway, and get him breathing again, he might have a chance. One thing is for sure. There's no way to work on him inside the truck.

"We've got to get him out of here," I announce, pulling out of the cab.

"We can try," the EMT says. "But if the truck starts to fall, that will probably be the end of it."

I stand back while two large firemen brace themselves against the front of the truck to hold it upright. A third crawls under and starts to pull the limp body out through the shards of the driver's side window.

As the surgical intern on the helicopter rescue team, my job is to stabilize and transport critically injured patients from the scene of an accident to the hospital trauma room, to bring them back alive. But I am only in the first weeks of the practice of medicine, and most days my judgment is clouded by what I don't know, haven't seen, and can't imagine handling. My greatest fear every time I go out is that I will fail to do something that needs to be done to save a life and, because of my error, I will lose a patient in flight.

On the first day of our emergency room rotation our chief resident instructed us in the fundamental dos and don'ts of practicing in the field.

"Never bring back a dead body," Dr. Z told us. "If you bring back a dead body, it's going to be here for hours, just taking up a room. There won't be any family around to claim it. No one will know who it is or where to send it."

Thousands of complicated "what ifs" had been streaming through my head the night before my first in-flight rotation. Is it better to attempt a subclavian (under the clavicle) or a femoral (in the groin) line? How do we put in a chest tube out in the field? When do we bypass the trauma room and go straight to the OR? It never occurred to me to worry about the patients who were already dead, how to dispose of them, whether to load them into the top rack or bottom or leave them behind. It hadn't sunk in that some patients might actually die while we were en route or shortly after we arrived and what we would do if that happened.

"So, what *do* we do with the body?" another intern asked.

"Just leave it there," Dr. Z answered. "That's somebody else's problem. Not yours. But if you bring it back here, you're going to catch hell. Now let's talk about how to intubate a trauma patient."

For all the internal debating I'd done trying to establish best practices on the go, it turned out that establishing an airway was one of the few life-saving maneuvers we would perform regularly in the field. The patient could die or sustain irreparable brain damage from lack of oxygen if this procedure was not done correctly. We were all familiar with the basic technique. Some of us had practiced it in the operating room on anesthetized patients or on the elderly who suffered cardiac arrest on the wards. But wherever we were, up till now, there had always been someone more senior looking over our shoulders, acting as a safety net, guiding us, steering our hands more to the right or left, directing us to pull harder with the laryngoscope or let up.

Now we were about to go out into the streets, where, for the first time, a patient would be depending on our skills alone for their very survival.

"If you're going to intubate someone, do it nasally," Dr. Z said, holding the tube up for demonstration. "You have to protect the cervical spine at all times. That means maintaining inline traction. Unless you know for sure that a person doesn't have a broken neck, you have to go through the nose, not the mouth."

I looked from Dr. Z to the tube and back again, taking in his instructions. There was no mannequin, no corpse, no one walking us through the steps. There was just Dr. Z and this tube with a ring trigger held high for all to see. Until then, I had only seen nasal intubations attempted under the most controlled circumstances by an anesthesiologist.

It was a skilled maneuver, one that took years of practice to master. I tried to envision how I, an inexperienced intern, would blindly guide a tube as thick as my index finger down a person's nose, past their tonsils, through the vocal cords, and into the airway. I could see myself in the middle of a freeway at rush hour on my hands and knees, bending over the bleeding and bruised face of an accident victim, working the tube like a divining rod and willing it to find the trachea.

But this was no place for uncertainty or doubt. In the hierarchical system that defined surgery residency, Dr. Z made the rules and we interns followed them. This technique would work because Dr. Z had said it would. After a fleeting moment of incredulity, I chased the possibility of failure from my mind and incorporated his words as gospel.

"Don't try to do too much out there," he said. "Secure the airway. Make sure there are two working IVs. Stop any obvious bleeding. That's it. The idea is to scoop and run. Load the patient and get back here."

HELICOPTER AMBULANCES are one more instrument in the trauma care toolbox that allow critically ill trauma victims to be treated faster. But they don't just move a patient from scene to hospital. They bring skilled personnel such as nurses and paramedics to the site of injury to begin treatment with intravenous fluids, drugs, and blood. Patients are then evacuated to trauma centers, where surgeons who have been briefed during the flight are prepared to operate immediately if necessary.

The air ambulances of today are a legacy of military medicine rooted in the history of transporting the wounded from geographically remote locations to hospitals during times of war.

THE FIRST HELICOPTER RESCUE arose as an improvised solution to a nearly impossible task. In 1944, a small reconnaissance aircraft piloted by an American and carrying three British soldiers was gunned down in a rice paddy behind enemy lines in Burma during World War II. There was no way to access the crash site by ground and no available airstrip nearby. Army commanders had numerous factors to consider and decisions to make in coming up with a plan to get the men out, finally deciding their best chance was to send the helicopter in.

Which helicopter to choose was not an issue. There was only one.

The Sikorsky YR-4B was a military version of the first crop of mass-produced helicopters introduced in 1934.[1] Helicopters were so new to the world that the first army helicopter pilots had to be trained at the Sikorsky plant in Bridgeport, Connecticut.[2] The YR-4B was, not surprisingly, a primitive aircraft, once described as a "flying shoebox with windows." The cockpit, a cocoon of Plexiglas panels joined by aluminum seams, had just enough room for a pilot and one passenger. The helicopter had no radio, instruments, or lights.[3] The fuselage was a flimsy frame of hollow steel tubes that had been welded together and covered by canvas. The piston-driven 200-horsepower engine could barely provide enough lift for a full load and was prone to breakdowns.[4]

This is the aircraft that Lt. Carter Harman was called upon to fly to Burma, six hundred miles away, on April 21, 1944, when the message was transmitted: "Send the eggbeater in."[5]

Harman did not fit the rowdy image of pilots assigned to the

First Air Commando Group, an independent cohort of narcissistic cowboys, irreverent to the point of insubordination.[6] The twenty-six-year-old was, by comparison, a slight, baby-faced choirboy. Before the war, he played the clarinet and studied music composition at Princeton. He had taken flying lessons, so he joined the U.S. Army Air Corps to avoid being drafted into the infantry and later volunteered to be in the first group of U.S. Army Air Forces pilots to train as helicopter pilots.[7] When it came to flying helicopters he was green, but so was everyone else in the first class to graduate from helicopter school only six months before the Burma mission.

No one informed Harman that he would be attempting a high-risk rescue, the first ever by an American helicopter pilot. He was simply told to fly the helicopter to an Air Commando base in Burma. The YR-4B had a range of only a hundred miles and refueling stations were spotty, so Harman piled four cans of gas in the copilot's seat. Behind the seats, he loaded a canvas-covered stretcher that could be attached to the helicopter's exterior. Then he took off, solo, making short hops through a number of airfields, spending the nights at bases along the way. Only when he finally arrived in Abdereen, Burma, was Harman told that he was being sent into enemy territory to rescue the downed crew.

American planes had located the crash site and had been dropping supplies to the men below. Because the YR-4B could carry only one additional passenger, the plan was for Harman to ferry out one man at a time and drop him at a sandbar near a neighboring river. A small plane would pick them up from there and fly them to the nearest base.

Harman knew he was going to have to push the YR-4B's engine to its limits to be able to get the men out. The danger of the mission was heightened by the fact that the crash site was surrounded by Japanese troops. But Harman made it through and loaded the most seriously wounded soldier first. The YR-4B vibrated and redlined as Harman took off in the humid jungle air, but he made it to the sandbar.[8] He then returned and brought out a second wounded soldier, but this time when he reached the riverbank his engine "seized" as he landed and would not start up again. The strained engine had overheated, and the only thing Harman could do was to let it cool overnight and try to start up again in the morning. Luckily, the engine did restart the next day and Harman was able to evacuate the remaining wounded soldier and pilot.

So dangerous was the territory and precarious the aircraft that Harman was risking his life every time he stepped into the cockpit and started the engine. He spent several more weeks in the area and flew another fifteen rescue missions before a combination of damage to the helicopter and enemy invasion forced him to stop. His pioneering heroics not only earned him the Distinguished Flying Cross but also demonstrated that the helicopter could serve as a viable evacuation option when there was no other way to reach the wounded.[9]

A NEW GENERATION of helicopters, the H-13s, played a more prominent role in the Korean War, where the task of evacuating casualties to Mobile Army Surgical Hospitals was thwarted by rugged terrain and the lack of road and bridge infrastructure. The H-13s came newly staffed with both medic and pilot, but the lightweight metallic "grasshopper," initially designated as an observation aircraft, was not outfitted for the exigencies of evacuation.[10]

There was still no room inside for a stretcher, meaning that patients had to be carried on litter rings mounted along the side of the helicopter. This arrangement posed several problems. First, a wounded patient could not be monitored or treated in flight, as he was physically separated from the onboard medic. Second, the external litters left the patients exposed to both the weather, raising the risk for hypothermia, and enemy fire.

The 200-horsepower H-13s were underpowered and could barely lift a load of a pilot and two casualties and had no armor to protect the crew. They had no radios, internal lights, or instruments; that is, they were not equipped to fly at night or in bad weather.[11] The pilots well knew the H-13s' limitations, but getting that across to the troops in the field could be difficult. When forced to fly at night, pilots would have to use handheld flashlights to see the controls. The transmissions, bearings, fan belts, batteries, and spark plugs were vulnerable to wear and tear and prone to malfunction, sidelining portions of the fleet while spare parts could be scavenged.

Helicopter rescue was expensive and temperamental and exposed pilots, crew, and the wounded to the danger of enemy fire. But an H-13 could be airborne within three to ten minutes and could deliver a wounded soldier to an operating room within an average of an hour from the time of dispatch. Compared to ground transport, which could take hours or even days, it was a vast improvement.

Helicopter transport was also less traumatic to an injured body than traveling across rutted roads on a jeep. Once a patient was onboard, a trained medic could at least begin resuscitation with IV fluids and blood transfusion and provide basic wound care before liftoff, all of which improved survival odds. Proof that this rapid evacuation was working was the improved mortality rate for soldiers who made it to treatment in the Korean War (2.4 percent) as opposed to World War II (4.5 percent).[12]

By the cessation of hostilities on July 27, 1953, the first designated medevac helicopters with trained crews had transported almost eighteen thousand wounded, many of whom would not have survived without them.

But even with these compelling statistics, medevac rescues still needed a champion who would push for a fully outfitted aircraft designed for rescue operations. Dr. Spurgeon Neel, wounded in the Battle of the Bulge in World War II, knew firsthand what it was like to be an injured soldier waiting for help.[13] Trained in aviation medicine, he arrived in Korea at the tail end of the war to command the Thirtieth Medical Group, overseeing seven surgical hospitals, two evacuation hospitals, ground evacuation units, and the First Helicopter Ambulance Company.

"Casualties are a 'perishable commodity,'" Neel wrote. "A man dies in so many minutes, not over a distance of so many miles. Any measure that will reduce the time lag between wounding and treatment will reduce both the morbidity and the mortality of war wounds."[14]

The "grasshopper" had clearly demonstrated its potential in Korea, warts and all, but its shortcomings were obvious. Neel urged the army to take the next step and commission the design and production of a designated rescue helicopter—one with flotation gear for offshore evacuations, instruments that enabled missions at night and in bad weather, and an internal compartment that would accommodate litters and allow a medic to work on a patient.

After Neel's tireless advocacy, the army announced a design competition for a new medevac helicopter in 1954. A group of Medical Service Corps officers worked with engineers and transportation specialists to design the new fleet. After reviewing twelve proposals from six different manufacturers, army officials awarded the contract to the Bell Helicopter Corporation of Fort Worth, Texas.[15]

Bell produced the first prototype of the UH-1 Iroquois helicopter, the "Huey," in 1956.[16] This new chopper was something the grasshopper pilots could only have dreamed of when they were piloting the pint-sized H-13 across Korea. The 800-horsepower gas turbine engine of the new UH-1 could lift two thousand pounds and fly at a brisk 140 miles per hour for up to 115 miles. Even with a full crew onboard (pilot, copilot, medic, and crew chief) it could transport up to two patients at a time.[17]

The call sign DUSTOFF was selected for medevac radio transmissions—a most fitting name, as helicopters blew dust on anything and anyone close to a landing zone.[18] Soon the term "dustoff" became synonymous with the Vietnam-era medevac helicopter.

As amazing as the new machine was, one thing it was not was bulletproof. Under the Geneva Convention, ambulances, hospitals, and the personnel staffing them, marked by the international symbol of a red cross on a white background, are to be treated as neutral in armed conflicts.[19] In Vietnam, however, that convention was not always respected. Some soldiers believed the red cross did nothing more than give Vietnamese snipers a clear target to aim at.

As former medevac pilot Paul Mercandetti explained, the army experimented with how to get the red cross message across to the enemy. "At first, we had just a red cross on a green helicopter. They shot at us. So we added a white border to make it more visible. They shot at us. So we added a white square to make it even more visible yet. And then we enlarged the square. Each time we lost an aircraft, they kept changing the cross to make it more visible."[20]

There was no such thing as a safe landing zone when picking up wounded from the scene of battle. Pilots might be forced to land during active firefights or be ambushed by sniper fire, and their lives were almost always in danger. They could request escorts from combat planes and helicopter gunships, but at some point they were left on their own. They were exposed on approach, in a hover, and in an improvised landing zone. Because pilots were at such high risk of injury or death in Vietnam, solo flights were banned so that if the pilot was hit, a copilot would be available to take over. Flying at night or in bad weather only added to the risk.

On top of the ambient dangers of being in a war zone, the do-or-die attitude of the pilots themselves, a sort of humanitarian machismo, added to the risk. Helicopter pilot Major Charles Kelly, who became commander of the Fifty-Seventh Medical Detachment in 1964, helped establish the mindset. Kelly insisted on stationing two medevacs as close to the action as possible and manned a helicopter in the Delta at Soc Trang, sixty miles southwest of Saigon.

Known as "Crazy Kelly," he had a rule for the young pilots who worked in his command: The wounded came first, and that meant no one refused a mission.[21]

Kelly also pioneered night missions to facilitate getting the wounded to hospitals as quickly as possible.

But Kelly never asked his men to do anything he himself wasn't willing to do. On July 1, 1964, a request came in for a medevac to evacuate wounded near Vinh Long. As Kelly skirted the area, the Viet Cong opened up on the Huey. The landing zone was in enemy territory, and the enemy was not going to let him in. He established radio contact with the unit on the ground and was told to back off because it was not safe to land.

"When I have your wounded," Kelly answered as the medevac took more hits.

As he started to set the helicopter down, the helicopter suddenly pitched up and fell over on its side, its rotors digging into the ground. Kelly had been shot in the heart through an open door, the first DUSTOFF pilot to die in Vietnam. As news of Kelly's death spread, praise flowed from all whose lives he had touched—the wounded he had saved, the pilots he had trained, his colleagues and superiors. Kelly's philosophy was not buried with him. Every new medevac pilot learned of his fearless legacy. *Fly the next mission. Now.*[22]

As the U.S. strategy shifted from advising the South Vietnamese to directly engaging in combat, the number of American troops increased from 23,000 in 1964 to 184,000 in 1965. The number of medevac units grew steadily to match the troop buildup, and by early 1966 there were four medevac detachments in Vietnam, each of which had twenty-five helicopters.

Bell Helicopter continued to make improvements to the Huey. In 1965 it introduced the upgraded UH-1D, which had larger-diameter rotors that enabled greater lift. This new version could carry up to fourteen passengers and nearly four thousand pounds of cargo.[23]

As the American ground forces increased, they penetrated deeper into the dense triple-canopy jungles of South Vietnam.[24] The combination of the rugged terrain and the dense vegetation added a new layer of difficulty to the medevac missions, as it was almost impossible to hack out a landing zone quickly and without exposing troops to enemy fire.

The time had come to roll out the Breeze hoist, a cable that could be lowered and attached to a wounded soldier. Capable of lifting six hundred pounds, the hoist was mounted inside the top of the cargo compartment and then swung out on a rotating arm that extended well clear of the landing gear. Several working attachments could be hooked to the hoist, such as a vest that could be strapped onto a wounded soldier or a metal litter for the more seriously wounded, but both tended to get hung up in the dense foliage when it was lowered through the trees.

The "jungle penetrator," a device specifically designed to penetrate the thick jungle canopies, arrived in the summer of 1966. The core was a three-foot-long, bullet-shaped body with a point on the lower end that could push through the trees vertically. Three hinged metallic slats were kept in a folded position as the hoist was lowered. When the penetrator reached the target below, the slats were folded down for the injured soldier to straddle while he was harnessed to the chair.[25]

While the hoists enabled the evacuation of wounded that might not otherwise be accessible, these missions exposed the pilot and his crew to additional hazards. A hoist mission required the pilot to stay in a high hover for as long as it took to retrieve the wounded, making the helicopter a visible and vulnerable target.[26]

While the hoist was in progress, the pilot had to concentrate on keeping the Huey totally still—a challenge in wind gusts or during firefights. The pilot could not see the hoist as it was lowered beneath the Huey or steer it around obstacles. These missions always took longer than a landing for a patient pickup and exposed the aircraft to enemy fire.

In January 1969, pilot Paul Mercandetti undertook a rescue mission that required two men to be evacuated by hoist. The first patient was pulled up without encountering any enemy fire. On the second pickup, however, all hell broke lose as Mercandetti hovered above the trees and dropped the jungle penetrator. He was taking direct hits into the belly of the helicopter, each shot echoing like popcorn popping. Then the instrument panel exploded, leaving the hoist jammed in the lowered position with the patient loaded, so he had to climb higher to pull the wounded man clear of the trees.

More fire was coming as the helicopter lost oil, fuel, and hydraulic pressure, but the Huey was still airborne. The first patient who had been loaded was shot through the floor of the fuselage, bullets hitting both testicles. With fuel pouring from the tanks, soaking the patient below, Mercandetti made it to an army base, where he gently lowered the patient, still clinging to the hoist, and set the chopper down beside him. Mechanics counted over fifty bullet holes in the floor of the helicopter, which was so damaged it could not be repaired.[27]

Over 496,000 medevac missions were flown from 1962 to 1973, and over 900,000 patients evacuated, but these impressive results were not without sacrifice. Approximately two hundred pilots and crew were killed in the line of duty and countless others wounded, and two hundred medevac helicopters were downed by enemy fire.

BECAUSE OF THE SUCCESS of medevacs in Vietnam, the National Highway Transportation and Safety Board offered matching funds in 1966 for states that wanted to test the feasibility of civilian helicopter rescue. One of the more successful community based programs was the Coordinated Accident Rescue Endeavor —State of Mississippi (CARE-SOM) program, in which three fifty-mile operational zones (Hattiesburg-Greenville-Tupelo) were set up. During a six-month period from 1969 to 1970, 1,306 missions were flown, 664 of which were classified as medical emergencies. Like the other handful of trial programs throughout the country, the CARE-SOM program demonstrated that running a civilian helicopter rescue operation was feasible and safe, although logistical issues presented some sizable obstacles. One of the reasons DUSTOFF had been so successful was that the U.S. Army had streamlined communications, allowing prompt dispatch of helicopters and communication, with physicians and staff on the receiving end. In the civilian world, communication between first responders, the helicopter crew, and the hospital destination remained a challenge.

Civilian helicopter programs continued to evolve in innovative ways that spread the costs and capitalized on existing expertise. In 1967 the University of Maryland's Shock Trauma Unit at Baltimore built a helipad that was initially used by the military to transport trauma patients. In 1968 the Department of Transportation provided a grant for enlarging the helipad, and by 1969 the Maryland State Police were transporting trauma victims from around the state to the trauma unit.[28]

In 1970 the Military Assistance to Safety and Traffic (MAST) program was launched from Fort Sam Houston in San Antonio, Texas. The fifteen-unit program flew H-model Hueys to evacuate civilian trauma patients to nearby trauma centers. Medevac advocate Spurgeon Neel helped establish the MAST program.[29]

In remote and difficult-to-access geographic areas, such as mountainous regions, helicopter rescue made sense, especially in the winter when road travel was hazardous or prohibited altogether. In 1972 St. Anthony's Hospital in Denver, Colorado, established the first civilian hospital-based medical helicopter service.[30] In cities that had large land areas and major traffic problems, such as Los Angeles and Houston, helicopter rescue would prove to be a huge advantage.

By 1980 there were 32 medical helicopter programs flying 17,000 patients in the United States. By 1990 this figure had ballooned to 174 programs evacuating 160,000 patients.[31] Today there are over 272 air ambulance services across the country, evacuating 650,000 patients a year.[32]

KNEELING OVER MY PATIENT in the middle of the night, I realize I am about to enter territory that extends beyond Dr. Z's brief orientation. Because of the injury, the excessive bleeding and probable transection of the upper airway, I can't insert a breathing tube through the mouth or the nose. The only thing left is a tracheostomy, a surgical airway placed through an incision in the neck.

My first tracheostomy should have been performed in a brightly lit operating room with a complete set of instruments, a cautery, and suction. An attending surgeon should have been assisting me while an anesthesiologist controlled the ventilation, administered oxygen, and monitored vital signs. But the opportunity to learn the technique gracefully has been supplanted by the challenge at hand.

I realize that in attempting a tracheostomy under these conditions I may violate more than one of Dr. Z's rules. I may be trying to do too much in the field, and if the procedure doesn't work, I could be forced to bring back a dead man who will needlessly clutter the trauma room while calls are made to the family, the medical examiner, and a funeral home. But regardless of Dr. Z's prior instructions, I know I cannot cut a person open and leave him in the middle of the road. This patient is coming back with me no matter what.

I turn to the flight nurse. "I need the Betadine, a scalpel, and a trach tube," I say.

"We don't carry trach tubes," she says.

A tidal wave of doubt floods my brain. Why don't they carry the tube I need? I have heard of punching through the trachea with a Bic pen. What else can I use?

"Then give me the endotracheal tube," I say.

The flight nurse crouches over the man's head, holding a flashlight while I palpate the landmarks. First I find the bulbous protrusion of the thyroid cartilage, the Adam's apple. Just below that, I locate the depression of the cricoid membrane. With no time to spare, I make an incision over it and use a hemostat to spread down to the trachea. I stick my finger in the hole to feel the airway, punch through the membrane, and spread the opening wider. I pick up the endotracheal tube and twist it into the opening, connect the ventilation bag, and start giving breaths. The chest rises and falls. The procedure is a success.

We waste no time loading the patient in the helicopter. As we land, I can still feel his pulse; I know I'm not bringing back a dead man. We unload "hot" and take him straight to the trauma room. The nurses draw labs. A transfusion is started. We get a CAT scan of his brain and assess his neurologic function. But by this time, the swelling in his brain is so great it is starting to force all the blood out of his skull. Within hours the blood flow will cease altogether and he will be brain dead.

My last duty is to tell his family the awful news. I find a white coat to put over my scrubs, streaked with blood, dirt, and grease, reeking of gasoline. I am still replaying the night's events as I walk into the quiet hush of the waiting room.

I tell them we've done everything possible but my patient, their loved one, is not going to make it, and I express my condolences.

I feel awkward among the crowd of mourners, like I have come up short on a fourth-quarter game-winning drive and let everyone down. Then I meet the waifish girlfriend wearing a blood-spattered tank top and cutoffs. Instantly, I feel a bond. Without her courage to run into the dark to find help, I would not have shown up to provide it. This night has tested us both, but we found out something about ourselves, about what we are capable of when no one else is around.

If it can happen on a dirt road in the middle of the night, it can probably happen anywhere.

5 » RESCUE WARRIORS

MITCHELL BROWN was a teenager when a blood vessel in his thirty-five-year-old mother's brain burst in the 1960s. The single mother and her two children lived in the Hill District of Pittsburgh, the impoverished center of the black community. The funeral home-run ambulances didn't respond to "dangerous" neighborhoods, so Mitchell called the police to take her to the hospital.

"Two white police officers refused to carry her—they said she was drunk. I carried her myself and put her in the paddy wagon. We took her to St. Francis Hospital. I never saw her alive again."[1]

The sole training of the personnel manning the Pittsburgh police wagons consisted of a ten-hour course in basic first aid. They were known for a "grab and go" mentality that provided little in the way of first aid at the scene and often resulted in disastrous outcomes.

Even the famous suffered.

Former governor David Lawrence was delivering a rousing campaign speech at the Shriner's Mosque in downtown Pittsburgh on November 4, 1966, when he collapsed from a cardiac arrest.[2] A nurse from the audience rushed to the stage and started CPR. She got a pulse back, providing a brief spark of hope that Lawrence might survive. And then a police wagon arrived on the scene to transport him to the hospital. Two attendants got out, lifted Lawrence onto a canvas stretcher, shoved him through the rear doors, and jumped back into the cab to take off.

The nurse barely managed to slide in beside the stretcher, but there wasn't enough room in the cramped rear compartment for her to perform chest compressions. Deprived of oxygen en route, Lawrence arrived at the hospital with a severe anoxic brain injury and died seventeen days later.

Dr. Campbell Moses, Lawrence's physician, summed up the issue in one sentence: "We've got to learn to do better in first aid."[3]

In 1960 only four states had specifications for ambulance design, only six required standard training for rescue personnel, and less than half of all ambulance attendants had received even basic American Red Cross first aid training.[4] In the netherworld of 1960s prehospital emergency care the fates of Mitchell Brown's mother and David Lawrence were an all too common occurrence in many cities across the country.

PHIL HALLEN had seen firsthand what happened when ambulance transport went awry—the mistakes, delays, and the general neglect of pressing medical issues. These problems traveled with the patient to the hospital and might result in death. A self-described social reformer from Syracuse, New York, Hallen had worked as a part-time ambulance driver while in grad school.

"I saw how desperately untrained everybody was," he said.[5]

Hallen went on to study public health at Yale with an eye toward improving prehospital care. In 1960 he moved to Pittsburgh as a newly minted hospital administrator and got a firsthand look at the city's ambulance service.

"People came to realize this system was not only outdated, but medically dangerous and lethal," he said.[6]

Governor Lawrence's high-profile demise from inadequate prehospital care provided Hallen with a window of opportunity. Could he turn that unfortunate event into an opportunity to upgrade ambulance service? There was little doubt that the city was plagued by inadequate emergency services that hit the inner-city neighborhoods the hardest. In a broader sense Pittsburgh's racially segregated inner city was also suffering from a lack of businesses and jobs. In 1967, Hallen drafted a blueprint for putting unemployed men to work as trained ambulance attendants in the impoverished African American inner-city neighborhood known as the Hill District.[7]

His proposal hit at a time of volatile race relations across the United States. Just three years before, President Lyndon Johnson had signed the Civil Rights Act of 1964, prohibiting discrimination on the basis of race, color, religion, or national origin. Just two years before, the March on Selma took place and Congress passed the Voting Rights Act, which was designed to end discriminatory tactics at the voting booth.[8]

Riots spurred a rush to the suburbs by white middle- and upper-class families. With less commercial revenue, city tax bases dwindled and inner-city schools deteriorated. Detroit was particularly devastated by a five-day riot that resulted in forty-three dead, two thousand injured, 683 buildings damaged or destroyed, and numerous businesses burned or looted.[9]

By the time Pittsburgh's riots began in 1968, inner-city neighborhoods like the Hill District were awash in poverty, unemployment, crime, and poor housing.[10]

At the heart of social unrest was a lack of opportunities for African Americans. The United Black Front and other organizations were urging black men to remedy the problem by starting businesses and employing other black men. Hallen's plan to put young men of color to work was exactly the kind of program Pittsburgh's blighted inner city was crying out for. The only question that remained was how he would get the financial backing to get it off the ground.

NOT EVERYONE would have had the guts to paralyze medical colleagues with curare, the plant extract once used in poison arrows, but anesthesiologist Dr. Peter Safar did just that in an operating room at Baltimore City Hospital in 1956, an era before CPR existed.[11] He was conducting the medical experiment to document that mouth-to-mouth ventilation worked. Safar filmed firemen and boy scouts leaning over sedated volunteers breathing into their mouths while pinching their noses. With each breath the oxygen levels of the sedated volunteers rose to normal; they fell again whenever the mouth-to-mouth breathing was stopped.

Dr. James Elam had just published a paper showing that mouth-to-mouth breathing effectively delivered oxygen into another nonbreathing person, and no one had paid much attention. But Safar was a pioneering emergency care specialist and immediately recognized the potential of Elam's discovery. Having lost his twelve-year-old daughter to an asthma attack, he wanted to promote the technique as a way to revive people who had stopped breathing outside the walls of a hospital.

Three hundred thousand Americans a year suffered cardiac arrest outside the hospital, but there was very little to do for them in the field. Over 90 percent never made it to the hospital alive.[12] Doctors were desperate to find ways to keep these patients going until they could get to the hospital, where they would at least have a chance to survive. The lack of effective field resuscitation techniques was also holding back the evolution of ambulance services from mere transport vehicles to providers of outside-the-hospital medical care.

Safar jump-started prehospital resuscitation in 1960 when he had the vision to join the A for Airway and B for Breathing with the C for Circulation. That is, he coupled mouth-to-mouth breathing with another life-saving maneuver being developed across town at Johns Hopkins—compressing the chest and forcing blood out of a sputtering heart after cardiac arrest. This innovation earned Safar the moniker "the father of CPR."[13]

Safar provided another boost to prehospital care in Pittsburgh when he agreed to sign on as medical director for Hallen's inner-city ambulance service. Safar was a well-known opinion leader in emergency and intensive care unit (ICU) medicine, and having him on board branded the project as credible. He put Hallen in touch with Gerald Esposito, the president of the Pennsylvania Ambulance Association. Esposito had been looking for an outlet to pilot an upgraded ambulance service and thought the project had potential. James McCoy Jr., a founder of Freedom House Enterprise Corporation in the Hill District, a company designed to foster African American businesses, lent the project community support and a name. Hallen, Safar, and McCoy connected with Moe Coleman, an aide to Mayor Joseph Barr who agreed to provide the last piece of the puzzle—a $100,000 contract between Freedom House and the City of Pittsburgh to provide ambulance services.

And just like that, a coalition was formed that virtually guaranteed that Freedom House Ambulance Service would become a reality.

WITHOUT NATIONAL STANDARDS, the competency of prehospital care relied on individual champions like orthopedic surgeon Dr. Joseph "Deke" Farrington in Chicago. He never intended to become an instructor in prehospital care, but when he saw the need he partnered with fellow orthopedic surgeon Dr. Sam Banks in 1963 to put together one of the first comprehensive training programs in prehospital care. This four-day course was given to the Chicago Fire Department's ambulance division. Farrington took the firemen to Cook County Hospital and walked them through the trauma center, one of the first in the nation.[14] He showed his trainees *The Four B's: Bleeding, Breathing, Broken Bones and Burns*, an instructional film on how to prioritize a trauma patient's treatment.

After thirty years of training first responders in Chicago and caring for hundreds of victims of orthopedic trauma, Farrington decamped for Lakeland Memorial Hospital in Minocqua, Wisconsin. He was expecting a slower-paced small-town practice, but he found just the opposite.[15] In the summer months the population in the small resort community swelled to thirty thousand as tourists drove their cars, trucks, motor homes, and motorcycles to town. Once again Farrington was hard at work taking care of car crash victims, but he found a "hair-whitening situation" in the ambulance service—a local hearse manned by untrained drivers. Patients were brought in without the benefit of basic first aid measures at the scene, such as splinting long bone fractures and securing a car to protect the spine during transport.

Farrington instituted the same type of training program in Minocqua that he had in Chicago and encouraged surgeons across the country to do the same in his article "Death in a Ditch," published in the June 1967 edition of the *Bulletin of the American College of Surgeons*. He painted an alarming picture of how crash victims were pulled recklessly from cars and loaded into the backs of ambulances for careening rides to the hospital.[16] "The responsibility for improving ambulance and rescue service rests with physicians," he wrote. "For too long apathy and a 'leave-it-to-others' attitude have prevailed."[17]

He preached the methodical and cautious extrication of crash victims, performing mouth-to-mouth resuscitation if indicated, taking whatever time was necessary to splint fractures. Patients with potentially injured spines needed to be secured by placing a collar around the neck and strapping the body to a backboard. These principles endure today in basic trauma patient stabilization.

AFTER MONTHS OF PLANNING, the inaugural class of Freedom House Ambulance Service began on November 1, 1967, at Presbyterian–University Hospital Emergency Room. The city had donated two secondhand police wagons and the funds to maintain them. Grants had been obtained to purchase basic equipment. Program recruiters had covered the neighborhood, going into the streets and pool halls and amassing a total of forty-three unemployed African American applicants. After a series of six interviews and psychological testing, twenty-five were selected to start.[18]

The Freedom House curriculum was, by Safar's design, more advanced and comprehensive than any previously conceived for prehospital providers. Phase 1, an intensive 142 hours of classroom instruction consisted of 35 hours of Red Cross first aid courses, 50 hours of anatomy and physiology, 30 hours of respiratory therapy, 20 hours of CPR training, 14 hours of medical ethics and professionalism, and 7 hours of defensive driving. Phase 2 provided an additional 172 hours of clinical training rotating through various departments in the hospital—the operating room, intensive care units, the morgue, the emergency room, and labor and delivery, along with lectures on clinical subjects.

The trainees received a frosty reception from the all-white hospital staff, some of whom assumed they were part of the custodial department; the patients were majority white as well. But the course instructors, including Safar and Dr. Nancy Caroline, gently pushed the racial barriers aside in the name of education. They brought their trainees into the operating room to learn how to place breathing tubes and intravenous lines and into the intensive care units to observe cardiac care.

After nine months or intensive training and exhausting exams, twenty trainees finished the program in July 1968 and began taking calls. In its first year the Freedom House program made 5,868 ambulance runs and transported 4,627 patients.[19]

THE EVOLUTION OF prehospital care depended on continued innovations that made it possible to save lives in the field. Cardiologists led the way in out-of-hospital resuscitation because in the 1960s most victims of cardiac arrest didn't make it to the hospital alive. Doctors had at least figured out why—ventricular fibrillation from coronary artery disease, a condition where the heart quivers ineffectively instead of beating. Inside the hospital, the heart could be shocked out of ventricular fibrillation with a defibrillator. The next step was figuring out how to get the heart beating again in the field.

Dr. Frank Pantridge of Belfast, Northern Ireland, was the first to convert a hospital defibrillator to a portable model that could be carried on an ambulance. He recruited a technician to help him convert the monster apparatus to a system that could run off of two 12-volt car batteries.[20] When he was done, the world's first "portable" defibrillator consisted of two car batteries, a static inverter that would convert battery power to electricity, and the 155-pound defibrillator.

The vehicle for Pantridge's mobile cardiac unit was supplied by the Belfast Cooperative Society's Women's Guild, which raised money to pay for unit number 331 of the Karrier Ambulance Fleet, aka "the cardiac ambulance," the first such unit in the world.[21] At first the oversized defibrillator was cumbersome to use, especially when it had to be hauled into upstairs bedrooms. There were reports of technical glitches such as loud pops and bangs emanating from the assorted components. At times the batteries failed to power the behemoth and the crew had to insert bare wires into electrical outlets to build a charge. By 1967, however, Pantridge was able to report that over a fifteen-month period all ten patients with ventricular fibrillation had been successfully resuscitated outside the hospital. Pantridge's landmark paper, published in the British medical journal *The Lancet*, described the technique of out-of-hospital defibrillation and showed that it was feasible.[22]

By 1968, Pantridge worked with bioengineer Dr. John Anderson to shrink the portable defibrillator to a more manageable seven pounds thanks to a miniature capacitor developed by NASA. The new iteration, the Pantridge 280, was housed in a bright red plastic box about the size of a six-pack, complete with a handle and docking base for recharging. A plastic-coated spiral cord connected a single paddle that was applied to the chest.[23] Six hundred units of this early model were sold in the United States as soon as it hit the market.

While Pantridge's work was not widely embraced in Britain, the *Lancet* article kicked off a wave of excitement through the cardiology community across the Atlantic and inspired a wave of mobile cardiac programs modeled after the "Pantridge Plan." It was as if American cardiologists had been poised and waiting for permission to start their own out-of-hospital resuscitation programs. Pantridge's success was all they needed to move forward with their own mobile cardiac units.

In Los Angeles, Dr. Walter Graf, working at Daniel Freeman Hospital in Los Angeles, echoed Pantridge's philosophy when he said, "If we could take advanced life support outside of the hospital walls, maybe we could save some of those who were being lost." He launched L.A.'s first mobile coronary care unit in 1969.

In Seattle, cardiologist Dr. Leonard Cobb collaborated with Seattle Fire Chief Gordon Vickery to establish Medic One.[24] In 1969 they purchased a twenty-four-foot mobile home complete with kitchenette from a Kansas company. Local firemen painted the imposing vehicle red and white and converted it into a replica of an intensive care unit room, complete with a central stretcher area, monitors, a defibrillator, and bags of intravenous fluid, along with medical supplies and drugs.[25] "Moby Pig" was big enough for several people to walk around in but bulged at the sides and was cumbersome to steer through narrow city streets. Still, it functioned as an innovative replica of exactly what it purported to be—an intensive care unit on wheels.[26]

The first year in service Medic One, staffed by physicians, responded to 630 emergency calls, 83 of which were cardiac emergencies. The next year, the first class of fifteen paramedics became the first responders after the law was changed to allow them to perform the required medical care in the field. But Medic One was much more than a well-staffed ambulance company. As a result of the elevation in on-scene medical expertise, more critical patients were making it to the hospital alive.

Medic One made it possible, not only to save cardiac patients, but also to rescue severely injured trauma patients who might have died at the scene. In 1983, Dr. Michael Copass and his colleagues published their experience treating patients who jumped from Seattle's Aurora Bridge. Jumps from extreme heights were almost uniformly fatal, resulting in collapsed and bruised lungs, cracked spleens and livers, and pelvic and femur fractures. Before Medic One existed the survival rate was less than 10 percent.[27] After Medic One the survival rate tripled. Paramedics out in the field were controlling airways, infusing intravenous fluids, and supporting blood pressures with medications, routine procedures by today's standards. But when the first waves of trained medics were hitting the streets, the procedures performed and the lifesaving results were nothing short of miraculous.

By the 1970s the idea of a trained prehospital workforce made up of EMTs and paramedics had gained traction. What physicians quickly found out was that you did not have to be a trained medical doctor or nurse to save a life in the field. All anyone needed to do was look to the role that medics had played in Vietnam to get a sense of what these new workers, the future EMTs and paramedics, were capable of. The range of clinical skills varied from taking vital signs and starting IVs to placing breathing tubes and putting in pacemakers.

"Ask any ten people for a definition of a paramedic and you're likely to get eleven answers—even if you ask ten paramedics themselves," said Dr. Nancy Caroline, an instructor for the Freedom House program known for riding with the medics in the streets of Pittsburgh.[28] In 1975, Dr. Caroline drafted a fifteen-module course that became the pioneering textbook *Emergency Care in the Streets*, a distillation of the Freedom House curriculum.[29]

Today EMTs and paramedics are essential first responders who rush to the scene of emergencies along with police and firemen.

And just like any other first responders, they put themselves in harm's way.

On September 11, 2001, within an hour of the first plane crash, twenty-three EMS supervisors, twenty-nine advanced life support units, and fifty-eight basic life support units were dispatched to the World Trade Center.[30] By the end of the day four hundred EMS personnel were on the ground. It is a well-known fact that a large number (341) of New York City firefighters and police officers died in the line of duty on that day. Eight EMS providers died too—four paramedics, three EMTs, and one volunteer ambulance dispatcher—a sober reminder that the men and women who provide medical care in the field put their lives on the line every day to save ours.[31]

OVER TIME THE SKILLS and professional demeanor they had worked so hard to acquire made Freedom House the preferred ambulance service for the most critical patients. At the peak of the program, a staff of thirty-five was running five ambulances throughout Allegheny County.[32] For the unemployed young men who joined the Freedom House program, the program had provided direction and hope just as intended.

"It was a real treat to be away from crime and other things that were going on in that area," recalled George McCary III, a 1968 graduate of the program. "To be able to go to work and actually help people . . . That's a big uplift whenever you have people praise something you do."[33]

Ultimately, the city decided to reform its own police ambulance program rather than subsidizing Freedom House any longer, and in 1975 the program was shuttered. In seven years of existence these trained emergency technicians, the forerunners of today's EMTs and paramedics, had set new standards for excellence in prehospital care and answered over forty thousand calls.[34]

Yet Freedom House had achieved much more. It had empowered more than one disadvantaged American to dream of a future outside the Hill District. Mitchell Brown, who had to carry his critically ill mother himself to the police wagon, became an air force medic and was subsequently hired by Peter Safar to work at Freedom House. Brown later became EMS commissioner in Cleveland and then public safety director for Columbus, Ohio. He attributes much of his success to Freedom House.[35]

"The people in the community had a sense of pride in the quality of service we were providing them and so did we."[36]

TWO »
TREATMENT

6 » HURT

ON FEBRUARY 27, 2007, a crisp, sunny day in rural Montana, seventeen-year-old Katie Holland reported for her after-school job at the stables where she boarded her horse. An active member of the Montana Paint Horse Club, she'd been riding since she was six years old; the walls of her room were papered with awards and horse posters. Her assignment for the afternoon was to learn how to drive the skid loader, a compact tractor with a bucket on the front used for scooping piles of dirt, manure, and hay.

Katie watched as a coworker took a turn at the wheel, and then she hitched a ride in the bucket to a manure pile for more practice. But on the way, the tractor hit a bump in the road. The bucket heaved up, causing Katie's right leg to pitch out and wedge between the tractor's front wheel and the back of the bucket.

As the powerful tractor kept moving forward, Katie's right leg and half her pelvis were literally wrenched away from the rest of her body. She spilled out of the bucket and onto the ground, a mound of torn muscles and blood marking the spot where her leg was once attached.

A quick-thinking coworker shoved everything within reach—her barn coat, clods of manure, and handfuls of hay—into the cavernous wound and shoved her knee up into the socket to put pressure on the bleeding vessels while another worker dialed

9-1-1. Katie, in shock from the blood loss, was in the middle of a manure pile, ten miles from the nearest hospital. Her chances of survival as she lay on the ground were dismal and diminishing with each passing minute.

"SHOCK . . . THINK OF IT as a pause in the act of dying,"[1] R Adams Cowley said, and he would have known after operating on heart patients in the 1950s before heart-lung bypass had been invented.[2] By necessity, his patients had to be cooled down and their hearts stopped while he was working on them. Without a pump, blood couldn't circulate throughout their bodies, leaving his patients in a state of controlled shock.

Cowley would operate as fast as possible, restart the heart, and send his patients to the recovery room in stable condition. And then, hours or days later, the ones who had suffered the most blood loss and the longest operative time would crash. Their blood pressures cratered, organs started to fail, and nothing could change the one-way street to certain death.

The same pattern emerged with the severely injured. Surgeons revived patients with blood transfusions, then got them through operations to stop the bleeding and repair the damage, only to watch them spiral down and die days later.

In the window of time it took to stabilize a bleeding patient, fill their tank, and get blood circulating again, something was happening inside the body—a metabolic derangement that Cowley could not understand or correct.

CIVIL WAR-ERA SURGEON Dr. Samuel Gross's description of shock was remarkably accurate. He spoke of it as "a deep mischief lurking in the system" that leaves "the machinery of life unhinged."[3]

Heart surgeon Alfred Blalock at Johns Hopkins is credited for describing the syndrome we know today as shock in 1943 and setting out a basic framework for understanding the causes. In addition to hypovolemic shock—that is, shock due to low blood volume or dehydration—shock can be caused by severe infection, anaphylaxis, spinal cord injury, and severe heart dysfunction. Blalock preferred the term "acute circulatory failure," as it was more descriptive and distinguished the condition from previous confusing and misleading uses of the word.

Today shock is defined as "a state of inadequate tissue perfusion," meaning that there is not enough blood and therefore oxygen traveling to the cells in the body. As a consequence, vital functions are endangered and there are metabolic abnormalities and dangerous shifts in fluid balance. The classic clinical triad of shock is low blood pressure, a racing heartbeat, and confusion.[4] The problem sounds deceptively simple: *not enough blood circulating in the body*. But the clinical ramifications of the condition are complex and profound. Past a certain point, it is still, to this day, difficult to reclaim a person suffering from shock.

EVEN WHEN COWLEY could see shock coming, he was powerless to stop the physiologic mayhem. Still, he refused to believe the deaths were inevitable and he went looking for a solution.

Experiments with dogs provided the first clues to what was happening. When he withdrew enough blood to throw the animals into shock, about half their blood volume, they would recover if he returned the blood within an hour. But if the dog was left with a low circulating blood volume for longer than an hour, returning the blood later might stabilize the animal, but not for long. It too would eventually succumb to shock. Cowley now knew that time was a critical factor in resuscitation, but he still didn't know why.

In 1959, the U.S. Army awarded Cowley a grant to study shock in humans, which led to the first clinical shock-trauma unit in the country, headquartered in two rooms in the basement of the University of Maryland Hospital.[5] One room housed equipment to analyze a patient's blood—measuring electrolytes, acid/base content, serum protein, hormones, and enzymes and the concentration of red and white blood cells. The other room was outfitted with a hospital bed and monitors of every known configuration to capture a patient's vital processes—EKG monitors, blood pressure, rate and depth of breathing, and urine output.

He trained a cadre of doctors and nurses to stay at the patient's bedside around the clock to record vital signs and observations and to draw blood samples hourly rather than daily, as was done in the rest of the hospital. Cowley was throwing the biggest net he could devise around this strange beast known as shock. He was out to catch it in the act, take it apart, find its weaknesses, and, if possible, defeat it.

Cowley's team scoured the hospital for patients other doctors had given up on and moved them to what his colleagues referred to as the "death lab." But on the way to defining shock, he found out he could actually do something to treat the condition. Because he was drawing blood samples hourly, he was finding abnormalities in blood chemistries as they unfolded and treating them before they got worse. He corrected potassium levels that were too high and sodium levels that were too low. He treated high acid levels in the body, a condition known as acidosis, that was detrimental to overall physiologic function.

Cowley used the latest medical equipment available, anything he could scrounge from the hospital, including a breathing machine that was normally available only in the operating room. This allowed Cowley to treat low oxygen and high carbon dioxide levels by adjusting the ventilator's rate and oxygen level.

What Cowley had done, in effect, was to create the first surgical intensive care unit, a specialized area of the hospital that honed in on abnormalities before they set off a cascade of metabolic missteps from which a patient could not recover. And in the process he discovered that making minute adjustments to patients' physiologic and blood chemistry parameters was saving lives. Half the people treated in the death lab didn't die. They got better and went home. And the patients that showed the most improvement were trauma patients who were typically young, previously healthy, and free of chronic disease.[6]

Cowley had made considerable progress treating shock, but the condition still had a 50 percent mortality rate, even with the best available treatment. He had another idea, though. In a move that echoed back to his early experiments, he decided to prioritize the speed of resuscitation in an attempt to avoid the insult of shock in the first place.

"If I can get to you, and stop your bleeding, and restore your blood pressure, within an hour of your accident . . . then I can probably save you," he said. "I call that the golden hour."[7]

Treatment of injury was time-sensitive, and nothing drove that point home like the concept of "the golden hour." Future generations of trauma surgeons all around the world would adopt the concept. Providing treatment within that first critical hour after injury, before a patient bled out, before the body's predetermined biological processes set the scene for shock to take hold, was crucial to a patient's survival.

WHAT BECAME CLEAR to Cowley was that with the large number of trauma victims dying from injury—fifty thousand across the nation, and eight hundred in Maryland alone—instituting a system that could save at least half would be well worth the effort.[8] He believed every patient in Maryland, regardless of ability to pay or where they lived, was entitled to the best trauma care available, and in many cases their lives depended on it. In Cowley's world that meant getting patients to the University of Maryland Hospital as quickly as possible.

Cowley envisioned a system of specialized trauma care that would funnel patients from across the entire state to his trauma unit. When it came to getting support for his vision, however, he met resistance from all sides—from hospital administration, neighboring hospitals, and his own colleagues.

In the early 1960s the rule of the land was to "scoop and run" and deliver an injured patient to the emergency room of the nearest hospital. Trauma patients tended to come in at night and on the weekends. There might only be one nurse on duty in a small-town emergency room. She would have to send for a doctor and couldn't order any kind of treatment until he arrived. There might be no blood available for emergency transfusions. X-ray technicians and operating room personnel, if needed, would have to be called in from home. Cowley found these practices abhorrent. In his mind, people who might have been saved at his hospital were dying unnecessarily from lack of basic facilities.

"The God's truth is that most emergency rooms are awful. I get into trouble every time I say that . . . but it's true."[9]

True or not, Cowley was not going to have it easy getting through to hospital administrators, politicians, and other disenfranchised parties. Even the members of his own medical staff were scratching their heads and wondering, "Doesn't Cowley have enough to do fixing hearts? Why is he poking his nose into trauma?"

Trauma was the bastard child of the healthcare system, rarely viewed as a legitimate disease entity that required special equipment, techniques, and expertise. There were no specialized training programs. The operations were considered basic procedures that anyone who could hold a scalpel could do—stop bleeding, close holes, take out parts that were beyond repair, connect up the rest.

Junior surgeons-in-training manned big-city emergency rooms and fumbled around for hours trying to decide whether a patient needed to go to the operating room. They called an attending surgeon only if an operation was necessary. The supervising surgeon would wander in from home after the operation was under way, lean over the shoulder of the chief resident, and take a peek, asking if he was needed. And many times he didn't bother to scrub in.

Now that Cowley, a well-trained surgeon, and a highly respected heart surgeon at that, had taken an interest in the injured and was calling attention to the existing deficiencies, he wasn't exactly the most popular man in the room. Disrupting the status quo almost always leads to discord, even if it meant saving lives.

Cowley became an army of one waging a war against trauma.

COWLEY WAS UNABLE to persuade the hospital to fund a dedicated shock-trauma unit. In the meantime, he continued to build his team and work toward improving the care of the severely injured. He collaborated with anesthesiologist Dr. T. Crawford McAslan to implement aggressive ventilator therapy to treat shock lung, a type of lung failure that developed in patients who had received numerous blood products.[10]

He recruited nurse Elizabeth Scanlon to work as his research assistant in the death lab in 1961, serving as both a sounding board and a collaborator. The two continued to collect data demonstrating that if they could get to a trauma patient within the "golden hour" and closely manage any complications of shock, they could save thousands of patients who would otherwise succumb to injury.

They considered the idea of configuring a tractor-trailer into a mobile operating room that could be stationed in trauma-dense areas of the city or dispatched to a scene. The operating room on wheels, similar to the Mobile Army Surgical Hospitals employed in Korea and Vietnam, would eventually become a reality in Iraq and Afghanistan when small mobile surgical teams were employed in Forward Resuscitative Surgery Systems.[11]

A more desirable option that arose was to transport injured patients by helicopter, but the expense was prohibitive for the fledgling trauma program. In 1963, however, Cowley was able to persuade the federal government to allow his trauma program to share helicopters with the state police. As part of the plan, Cowley would train state troopers as medics to man the helicopters.

In 1963 the federal Department of Transportation agreed to purchase helicopters for the state of Maryland to be shared in an innovative joint medevac and law enforcement program, the first of its kind in the country.[12]

But the feds threw in an added bonus for Cowley. Impressed with his plan for a centralized trauma unit, the Department of Health, Education and Welfare (HEW) awarded him $800,000 to fund half of a planned five-story building designed specifically for treating trauma patients and advancing trauma medicine. Under Cowley's plan, the first floor would be the admissions area, including an accident room with state-of-the-art equipment such as ventilators. This area would be staffed 24/7 by doctors and nurses. The second floor would include a trauma lab for running tests. The third floor was the operating room and recovery area. And the fourth floor was a twelve-bed intensive care unit with one-on-one around-the-clock care.

Surely the university hospital administration would be as inspired by Cowley's plan as the federal government was and pony up the other $800,000. But the hospital didn't have that much money lying around, and in order to fund the trauma institute, they would have to defund some other department, a very unpopular and unlikely move.

Academic and hospital politics effectively stalled the project for another four years. And during those years Cowley was vocal about the fact that people were needlessly dying on the streets of Baltimore and throughout the state of Maryland. He had a plan to save them, and the federal government had even endorsed it, but the University of Maryland was standing in his way.

In response, Cowley was accused of "empire building," trying to make a power grab by insisting on a standalone trauma center that would come entirely under his purview. But not everyone saw it that way.

"He's a brilliant creative genius," said psychiatrist Dr. Nathan Schnaper. "He's innovative and he's a pain in the ass."[13]

But that reputation didn't bother Schnaper a bit. He joined the shock-trauma team and stayed for over a decade.

The five-story trauma unit finally opened in 1969, six years after HEW had offered the seed money, but there were still bumps in the road. There was the political fallout when state troopers landed at accident scenes and loaded the patients into helicopters instead of allowing the local ambulances to take them. Physicians manning emergency rooms in community hospitals accused Cowley of stealing their patients and in retaliation held on to them.

The University Hospital refused to staff the shock-trauma operating rooms, requiring Cowley's trauma patients be transported out of the shock-trauma emergency room, down a hallway the length of a city block, and up seven floors to operating rooms in the main hospital for life-saving procedures.

"In one eight-month period I lost fifteen patients just trying to get them from here over to the main hospital and up to the operating rooms," Cowley seethed.[14]

In 1973, Governor Mandel issued an executive order that gave Cowley's trauma unit a new name and a whole lot more clout. It became the Maryland Institute for Emergency Medicine, funded as a line item in the state budget, and named Cowley the first director.[15] Cowley's vision of an integrated statewide EMS system of care funded by the state and linking first responders with ground and air transport and the Maryland Shock Trauma Center was on the horizon.

The battle for funding and territory was over.

OUR NATION'S TRAUMA CENTERS grew out of a complicated mix of wartime experience and policy decisions. In the late 1950s and early 1960s, the expertise to treat trauma victims began to flow back to the United States from the conflicts in Korea and Vietnam in the form of returning combat surgeons and medics. They had witnessed the necessity of trained prehospital providers and rapid ground and air transport, and the importance of treating shock. Civilian trauma care fed off of this military-based experience in city and county hospitals in large metropolitan areas championed by these veteran war surgeons.[16]

In Chicago in 1966, World War II veteran Dr. Robert J. Freeark and Dr. Robert J. Baker devised a central location at the city's Cook County Hospital for all trauma-related services, including dedicated critical care units for trauma patients. San Francisco General Hospital under the direction of Dr. William Blaisdell was another of the first trauma centers.

In a radically forward-thinking move for the time, Illinois funded a combined regional trauma program and statewide EMS system in 1971 with state and federal funds from the National Highway Safety Act of 1966.[17] Cook County trauma surgeon Dr. David R. Boyd, who had trained under R Adams Cowley, was recruited to draft a statewide system of trauma centers with supporting emergency medical services.[18]

On the policy front, the National Academy of Sciences had made its vivid pronouncement in 1966: An unchecked epidemic of trauma was ravaging the population. But no matter how severe the problem, it would be decades before there was a national coordinated effort to solve it. The federal government would continue to publish periodic reports on the state of trauma, but the lack of consistent federal funding undercut the development of a national trauma system.

Studies performed around the country made clear that having trained surgeons on staff was not enough to save the injured. What was needed was a trauma system with organized transport to trauma centers where surgeons were already in the hospital, experienced triage nurses in emergency rooms, blood banks that operated twenty-four hours a day, and an operating room that was available around the clock with trained personnel.[19]

Despite irrefutable evidence that trauma systems saved lives, trauma systems were slow to develop.[20] Subsequent reports by the National Research Council (1985) and the Institute of Medicine (1999) determined that even though trauma systems were having a positive impact, the trauma epidemic continued to rage and insufficient resources were being devoted to a public health threat of this magnitude.[21]

Being treated at a Level I trauma center lowers the risk of death by 25 percent, but not all trauma victims have immediate access to this highest level of trauma care.[22] In fact, nearly 45 million Americans are still not within an hour of a Level I or II trauma center.[23] The lack of emergency care and trauma centers has a disparate impact on the poor and those in rural areas, who are geographically more distant from trauma centers. While forty-two of the fifty states had established statewide trauma systems as of 2010, government funding of trauma centers is always at risk of being cut, and in some areas of the country access to trauma care has been shrinking. Between 1990 and 2005, 339 trauma centers closed, not because they weren't needed and not because they weren't doing a good job. They closed because of cost.[24]

KATIE'S COWORKERS KEPT talking to her, asking questions about where she had ridden her horse that day, as they waited for help. When EMS arrived, paramedics applied pressure to her open wound and started IVs. Katie's face was drained of color, her extremities cool; her heart was racing and her blood pressure was barely registering. Knowing they could lose her any moment, the medics didn't waste a lot of time at the scene. Katie watched as the lights above the rear doors of the ambulance came in and out of focus. She lost consciousness as the medics loaded her into the ambulance.

The crew radioed ahead to Deaconess Hospital in Bozeman to prepare an operating room. A surgeon with trauma experience happened to be on call on that day and met Katie's stretcher as she was rolled in. A rapid anesthetic was administered while the trauma team transfused her with blood. Then, once Katie was asleep, the surgeons picked out the hay and debris that her co-workers had used to pack the wound, tied off bleeding blood vessels, and repacked the wound with sterile gauze.

At the same time that the Bozeman doctors were working to stabilize Katie, the emergency room was calling for a helicopter to fly her to the nearest trauma center, which was 550 miles away: Harborview Hospital in Seattle, Washington, one of the elite trauma hospitals in the United States.

Up to that point Katie had been saved by a series of quick-thinking first responders, people on the front lines who were trained in first aid (Katie's coworker); emergency response (the ambulance EMTs); and the management of trauma victims (her surgeon at Deaconess). But Katie would need more to survive—the very best trauma care available at the hands of experienced surgeons, orthopedic surgeons, plastic surgeons, and rehabilitation specialists that could only be found at one of the best trauma hospitals in the country.

AS MUCH AS WHAT HAPPENED to Katie might seem like a freak, one-of-a-kind accident, it has actually happened enough to have a name. Traumatic hemipelvectomy, a severing of half the pelvis and the leg from the body, is seldom survivable, but for those that do make it, the injury has been described as catastrophic, mutilating, and life altering.

Traumatic hemipelvectomy leaves behind one of the largest open wounds a trauma surgeon will ever encounter in a living patient, one that many describe as "overwhelming." Pelvic organs like the bladder and rectum are frequently laid bare in the wound and damaged. Muscles are shredded. Nerves are snapped. The spurting ends of large blood vessels like the iliac artery and vein portend an impending fatality unless quickly controlled.

But people do survive this injury. As of 2005 there were a reported sixty-five survivors described in the medical literature.[25]

The chances of survival, a dismal 20 percent, reflect the fact that most victims succumb quickly to massive hemorrhage at the scene of the injury and never make it to the hospital alive.[26] Over the last two decades the number of reported survivors has been increasing due to improved prehospital care and rapid transport to hospitals, but the mortality rate remains extremely high.

Even after patients have made it through the initial threat of bleeding to death at the scene, their lives are still at risk for weeks. They have almost certainly been in shock and at risk for organ failure but are also prone to complications like pneumonia and invasive infection.

THE 415-BED Harborview Hospital in Seattle is the only Level I trauma center for the four-state region of Washington, Alaska, Montana, and Idaho. A Level I center provides the highest level of care, with twenty-four-hour availability of trauma surgeons, neurosurgeons, orthopedic surgeons, plastic and reconstructive surgeons, radiologists, a fully staffed operating room, and state-of-the-art intensive care units manned by experienced nurses and respiratory therapists. A Level I trauma center, in other words, brings together all the expertise a trauma patient could possibly need at the time that she most needs it.

The average car crash victim with brain, abdominal, and extremity injuries will have several trauma surgeons, a neurosurgeon, and an orthopedic surgeon evaluating and working on her at the same time. The Harborview trauma team, known as the Blue Wave because of the swarm of doctors and nurses attired in blue scrubs that descend on a new trauma patient, evaluates over five thousand trauma patients a year, an average of fifteen per day.

When Harborview trauma surgeon Dr. Hugh Foy got the call from Bozeman, he knew Katie had severe injuries.

"The surgeons there are very good," he said. "They don't send simple injuries."[27]

Foy was a thirty-year veteran of traumatic injuries of every kind, but he had never seen an injury quite like what he uncovered in the operating room at Harborview when Katie arrived. He watched as layers of gauze were unwrapped for several minutes, finally revealing an open wound that extended from her bladder and vagina around her vacant hip socket and ended at her sacrum. Hay and horse manure were still stuck in the crevices of the exposed organs and muscles.

Like many severe injuries that Foy deals with, there was nothing in any surgery textbook that could provide instructions for how to deal with an injury like Katie's. The first trip to the operating room and the daily trips over the next five days were to keep picking out contaminated debris and scraping away any muscle or tissue that had died. On the sixth day, a colostomy was performed to divert stool away from the wound and help keep the area clean.

Over time, Foy and his team were able to get the wound closed using extra-thick Alloderm, a bioprosthetic material made from donated human skin that comes in sheets several millimeters thick. All the native cells are removed, leaving a collagen scaffolding that a patient's own cells populate over time.[28]

The reconstruction of Katie's abdominal wall and pelvis required twenty trips to the operating room, two weeks in the intensive care unit, and another forty-nine days in the hospital. Once Katie's wound was closed, she was transferred to the rehabilitation unit, where she spent two hours a day learning to walk again, first with a walker and later with forearm crutches. The prosthesis she sometimes wears has three joints—hip, knee, and ankle—and attaches to her torso with a bucketlike device that she straps around her waist. After leaving Harborview, she continued rehab at home in Bozeman, and after months of intense training and exercise Katie was able to attend her high school graduation and walk across the stage to accept her diploma.

In 2010, Texas saddlemaker Randy Bird, himself a paraplegic after a car crash, crafted a special custom-made saddle for

Katie.[29] It was adorned with silver accents, hand-engraved turquoise flowers, and Katie's initials. More importantly, it was fashioned with a high back and a wraparound leather band to hold her securely in place so she could ride again.

IN 1989, THE eight-story R Adams Cowley Shock Trauma Center at the University of Maryland, the only freestanding trauma hospital in the country, was opened. Today the facility has grown to 120 beds, including 50 ICU beds, ten operating rooms, and a Trauma Resuscitator Unit. In 2014, the trauma center admitted 8,265 patients, 20 percent of whom arrived by helicopter. The chances of surviving an injury if you are brought there today are 97 percent, a considerable upgrade from the 50-50 chances in the death lab a half-century ago.[30]

The state of Maryland trauma system has expanded from a two-bed death lab to a fifty-hospital network with eleven trauma centers, 450 ambulances, eleven helicopters stationed in seven locations, and a $15 million communications system.[31]

R Adams Cowley wasn't always popular in the pursuit of his mission. He stepped on some toes. He was accused of grandstanding and empire building, but he shrugged all that off. The man had a vision of what it would take to save lives and pursued it with passion, and because he did there are thousands of people walking around today who wouldn't have made it otherwise. With each passing day, his legacy marches forward and more survivors are added to the list.

7 » THE COLOR OF BLOOD

All bleeding stops eventually.

It's one of those pithy truisms that a junior medical student, as fresh and unsoiled as her short white coat on the first day of clinical rotations, tosses back and forth in her mind until the phrase becomes embedded, indelible. This everlasting truth will stay with her forever, and twenty years into the future, when she has a mortgage and a kid to put through private school, she'll hear it again.

When it's after midnight and she's been at it for hours, peering into a belly with blood welling up from some hidden hard-to-get-to crevasse behind the junction of the pancreas and the duodenum, the site of a large vein with a million tiny side-branches, the familiar words will dance through her brain. *All bleeding stops eventually.* They will pop out of a groove made what feels like a hundred years ago and remind her that as tedious as it is to be rooting around for something that is next to impossible to find, especially in the middle of the night with a full schedule looming the next day, this too shall end.

She prays it will end for all the right reasons—because she tied off the spurting artery or leaky vein, because she plugged the hole with a wad of Surgicel and held pressure until her fingers cramped, because she sewed up the ragged edges of a ruptured organ—not because the red stuff came out faster than she could pump it back in, causing the entire system to crash like an over-loaded server tapped by one too many requests.

All bleeding stops eventually.

Please let it be because she found the hole and not because the heart gave out and failed like a gasping sump pump in an outdoor fountain when the water's been completely drained for hours. If the heart stops beating, whatever's left in the vessels will stop moving too, stuck in the large veins of the chest, abdomen, arms, and legs, where it will clot in place and never move again.

All bleeding stops eventually.

And when it does, it is either the excuse for a raucous celebration that echoes down the darkened hallways of the graveyard shift or the beginning of a very long night of regrets and missed opportunities to save a life.

BLOOD CIRCULATES through our bodies carrying oxygen to all our tissues and organs. They cannot function without it. We must have an adequate supply of red blood cells to stay alive. But our body's reservoir of blood is threatened by major injury—the greater the impact, the more bleeding one can expect. One of the worst things that can happen in trauma is that an injured patient bleeds so much and so quickly that he dies before anyone has a chance to fix what's wrong with him. Yet it happens every day.

It happens because an injury is so massive the bleeding can't be contained and the patient is gone before anyone has even thought to call 9-1-1. It happens because someone is injured in a remote location, bleeding until the tank is drained. It happens because doctors and nurses, even in the best of hospitals, can't control the source of bleeding in time.

Exsanguination is defined as "the act of draining a person, animal or organ of blood"—or, in medical jargon, "bleeding out."[1] When a trauma patient has lost more than half his blood volume, he is in the process of bleeding out. If he still has a heartbeat at the two-thirds mark, it probably won't last for long.

Of the approximately 5 million people who die around the world from trauma every year, at least a third bleed to death.[2] Massive hemorrhage is second only to traumatic brain injury as the cause of death from injury.

With battlefield injuries the numbers are particularly sobering. Ninety percent of soldiers who die with potentially survivable wounds bleed to death. That's 90 percent who could have healed up from everything else that was torn apart by a bullet, bomb, or grenade, except for the fact that too much blood was lost. For this reason alone, military surgeons have become experts at stopping bleeding, and luckily for us, they have passed that expertise on to the civilian world.

BEFORE THEY EVER laid eyes on the twenty-four-year-old soldier, the Forward Surgical Team in remote Afghanistan was notified of his critical condition and started to prepare.[3] The young man had been strafed with an AK-47, an assault rifle designed to kill with stunning efficiency. Multiple rounds struck his torso and legs, each two-inch bullet traveling at 2,350 feet per second, capable of piercing the metal of a car door and killing its intended target inside.

His surgeons were well acquainted with how bullets like these tear through the human body, leaving a meandering trail of destruction like a tornado through a trailer park. They also knew that if they could control massive hemorrhage, the most common cause of preventable death in combat casualties, they might be able to save a life. From the reports they were getting en route, the soldier was already sinking into shock, a lack of adequate circulation in the body from a massive loss of blood. His only chance at survival would be a flawless execution of the medical team's resuscitation game plan.

UP TO 16 PERCENT of patients who die from hemorrhage might have been saved if bleeding had been recognized earlier and treated effectively.[4] Undetected internal bleeding into the abdomen or pelvis usually accounts for most of these preventable deaths. But a trauma victim can also bleed to death from external hemorrhage, like bleeding from an arm or leg that no one manages to control in time. Applying a tourniquet, a ten-second procedure, might have saved him.

Armed with statistics such as these, trauma surgeons are starting to reshuffle the deck on priorities in resuscitation, particularly in combat. For the better part of a half-century, the "controlling bleeding" part has been the third priority in Advanced Trauma Life Support classes, behind airway and breathing problems, because these were considered the most immediate threats to life.

"Stop bleeding," however, is climbing the priority list thanks largely to the efforts of military physicians who discovered that most combat casualties die within ten minutes of being wounded, and usually from exsanguination.[5] In a one-year period, ten soldiers were dead on arrival to a Baghdad combat support hospital after isolated limb exsanguinations.[6]

The military's MARCH protocol (Massive Hemorrhage, Airway, Respirations, Circulation, and Hypothermia) now instructs army medics to stop external bleeding before doing anything else.[7] Direct pressure is applied first. If the bleeding continues and the source is an extremity, a tourniquet is applied above the site of bleeding.

Tourniquets fell out of favor and were shelved during World War II and Vietnam due to the concern over impairing the blood supply to a limb and damaging it further. But they have made a comeback based on a decade of combat experience in Iraq and Afghanistan.[8] The combat application tourniquet is a simple tourniquet that can be applied by a wounded soldier with the use of only one hand.[9] Applying a tourniquet before a patient goes into shock can improve survival by 90 percent. Because of the favorable results from using tourniquets, the morbidity of extreme blood loss, and the ease of use, they are becoming part of standard civilian EMS procedure once again, and some are suggesting that other first responders, such as police, carry them too.

Hemostatic bandages, like QuikClot Combat Gauze, are bandages impregnated with kaolin, an agent that accelerates the body's ability to form a blood clot and therefore stop active bleeding in a wound.[10] These bandages can stem bleeding in anatomic areas that cannot be easily compressed or controlled with a tourniquet, such as the axilla or groin.

Tracking down the source of internal bleeding will usually require a more in-depth investigation utilizing imaging studies such as a CAT scan or bedside ultrasound to try and pinpoint the body cavity and organ source. Even if the exact location isn't known, innovative solutions are emerging to compress internal bleeding until a wounded victim can make it to the hospital.

In the "medical version of Fix-a-Flat," a syringe full of small spongelike discs impregnated with a clotting agent can be injected into an open wound like a bullet hole in the abdomen.[11] The sponges expand to ten times their size within seconds to plug the wound and internally compress bleeding sites. This device, the XStat, is exactly the type of tool that could stabilize a soldier on the battlefield until he can reach a hospital. Approved by the Food and Drug Administration (FDA) in 2014, the XStat is now available in both the military and civilian markets.

BY THE TIME the young soldier arrived at the field hospital, his heart was in overdrive at 150 beats per minutes, his blood pressure dipping below 70 mm Hg, and his abdomen felt swollen and tight from the blood accumulating inside. Medics hung blood and plasma and rolled him into an operating room where surgeons stood scrubbed and gowned.

Simply inducing anesthesia, which causes dilation of the blood vessels, could be enough to collapse his cardiovascular system, so instead of the usual sequence of putting the patient under and then prepping and draping, the doctors reversed the order, prepping first, and then stood by. This way, if the patient crashed they could quickly open his abdomen.

As soon as the anesthetic drugs were given, the patient's blood pressure dipped further, prompting the surgeons to immediately open his abdomen through a midline incision. As they pressed the knife into the layers of the abdominal wall and through the peritoneal lining of the abdominal cavity, blood spurted out of the incision and across the drapes. The well-rehearsed team responded automatically to the profuse rush of blood, packing each quadrant of the abdomen with a fistful of sponges to stanch all possible sources of blood loss. Meanwhile, the anesthesiologist administering blood at the head of the table could catch up with the blood loss and hopefully stabilize the patient.

Despite the packs, the soldier continued to bleed from the right upper quadrant, where the bullet had blasted through his liver, shredding the trellis of blood vessels threading both lobes. During the bloodiest moments the surgeons were clamping and tying off large veins that dumped into the dome of the liver under the right diaphragm, finally slowing the torrent. The surgeons packed again, their eyes turning in unison to the monitors at the head of the table to watch as the patient's blood pressure inched above one hundred and into the normal range.

There were other injuries to contend with too—tears in the stomach, small intestine, and colon that had dumped unsterile gastric contents and stool into the belly, leaving a stew of bacteria, food particles, and freshly clotted blood. The surgeons took a damage-control approach, doing only what they had to do to stop the bleeding, close the holes, and wash out the abdomen. They cut out unsalvageable portions of intestine, stapled across the ends, and covered the abdominal opening with sterile plastic sheets.[12] The soldier's leg wounds were quickly cleaned, wrapped, and splinted, and he was taken to recovery.

The wounded soldier had received twelve units of fresh whole blood, twelve more units of packed red blood cells, thirteen units of plasma, five units of clotting factors, and a dose of recombinant Factor VIIa, a synthetic clotting drug, and for now he was out of shock and his blood count was near normal. His surgeons had controlled all sources of bleeding and contamination, and everything else that needed to be repaired could wait until he was more stable. Within an hour he would be transferred to a Level III Combat Support Hospital for definitive treatment.

The Forward Surgical Team had made all the right moves and could count this one as a victory.

EVERY YEAR, the blood banking system in the United States relies on the altruism of the 9.2 million individuals who donate 15.7 million units of blood.[13] Demands on the blood supply, up to 41,000 units per day, are on an upswing due to medical advances in cancer therapy and transplant surgery, along with the continued needs of trauma and burn patients. For example, at M. D. Anderson Cancer Hospital in Houston, two hundred units of red blood cells and six hundred units of platelets, on average, are administered *per day* to cancer patients.[14] But as reliable as the system has been in meeting the needs of modern healthcare, seasonal shortages during the summer months and winter holidays can still cause operations to be cancelled and treatments to be placed on hold until an adequate supply of blood is available.

TODAY WE TAKE for granted that if we need a blood transfusion, we can go to just about any hospital in America and get one, but that wasn't always the case. Getting the current blood-banking system off the ground required both convincing the American public that donating blood was safe and figuring out a way to collect and preserve blood. It took a war to spur the United States to take the lead in doing both.

While transfusions had been performed since the 1920s, the methods used in the United States for banking blood—that is, storing it for future use—came to fruition during World War II.

By the fall of 1940 Britain had officially been in the war for only a year, but things weren't going well for the Allies. The French had already surrendered, and the Germans were thrashing England with the largest sustained bombing campaign in the history of mankind, taking out air bases, strategic targets, and civilians with a ruthless show of force. The United States had not yet joined the war, and American doctors were trying to come up with a way to assist their British counterparts in treating wounded soldiers.

The U.S. military, anticipating that the country would soon be drawn into the war, had already appointed medical officers to investigate how blood could be collected, packaged, and transported for wounded soldiers overseas. There was no national donor program, and the availability of hospital-based blood transfusions was spotty throughout the country.

But there was a synergy building in New York City, the home of the Blood Transfusion Betterment Association, one of a handful of privately run blood services and the nation's first blood service. The top blood transfusion research program at Columbia Presbyterian Hospital, pioneered by surgeons John Scudder and Charles Drew, also happened to be in New York.

On June 12, 1940, leaders in the blood-banking community called a special meeting of the New York Academy of Medicine to discuss how to collect and ship blood to the Allied forces in Europe. The summit brought together representatives from the Blood Transfusion Betterment Association; the army surgeon general's office; top blood researchers from across the country, including Scudder and Drew; and scientists from commercial laboratories.[15]

During the meeting, Scudder first reported that he and Drew had been experimenting with preserving plasma. They had already prepared a small sample that a colleague had carried overseas, and the two had proven that plasma could be preserved for at least two months by refrigeration.[16] All in attendance agreed that plasma rather than whole blood should be shipped to the Allies in either liquid or dry form.

From the meeting, the Blood for Britain project was born—a program to collect blood from donors in the United States, separate and process the plasma portion, and ship it to the British Red Cross. Charles Drew was one of the foremost experts on banking blood and a logical choice to act as medical director of the Blood for Britain program. He agreed to return from Howard University in Washington, D.C., where he had recently taken a position, to head up the project.

One of his first moves was to standardize collection techniques in a central location. He made sure that only trained personnel collected blood, and he instituted strict quality controls on both donation and processing to decrease bacterial contamination.[17]

By 1941, Drew's plan for a model blood-banking system was up and running and he was named medical director of the Red Cross's pilot national blood plasma program. The Red Cross program initially produced dried plasma, plasma that had been converted into a powder form. Dried plasma did not require refrigeration and took up less space than liquid plasma, and was therefore easier to ship over long distances. Because it didn't need to be refrigerated, "the number-one lifesaving agent of the war" could be stored closer to the battlefield and reconstituted as needed.

Drew also promoted the donor program in novel ways, supervising the first mobile blood collection unit, the bloodmobile, for the Red Cross.[18] Blood for Britain, which operated for only five months, collected blood from fifteen thousand Americans to send overseas and was judged a resounding success.

In April 1941, Howard University recruited Drew back to Howard to become the chairman of surgery. His innovative work for the New York chapter of the Red Cross served as a template for the development of the American Red Cross's national blood bank.

After all he had achieved with the Red Cross, Drew was considered by many to be "the father of the blood bank," but he was a pioneer in another way too. Charles Drew was an African American physician in 1940, well before the civil rights movement, performing groundbreaking scientific research. The fact that he had earned a seat at the table with the preeminent blood researchers of the day and held the credentials to be included was a significant accomplishment given the limited opportunities available to African Americans at the time.

The Civil Rights Bill of 1957 guaranteeing voting rights to all citizens was still seventeen years in the future. Martin Luther King Jr.'s "I Have a Dream Speech" was twenty-three years away. How had Charles Drew, the son of a carpet layer and a teacher from Washington, D.C., managed to make his unlikely way through medical school and surgery residency and into one of the most prestigious universities in the country?

Amherst College in Massachusetts awarded Drew an athletic scholarship and served as his academic launch pad. He then attended medical school at McGill University in Montreal, Canada, where he first started working on treating shock and investigating techniques for fluid resuscitation with Dr. John Beattie, graduating in 1933.[19] He continued training at McGill while he applied to surgery residencies in the United States and finally accepted a spot at Howard University, the country's only black medical school at the time.[20]

After he trained to become a surgeon, the Rockefeller Foundation awarded Drew a two-year fellowship that paid for two years of graduate school at Columbia Presbyterian Hospital under the direction of the accomplished surgeon Dr. Allen O. Whipple. But in 1938, African American physicians were not permitted to treat white patients, so Whipple assigned Drew to work in Dr. John Scudder's surgical laboratory, where he conducted experiments in fluid balance, blood chemistry, and blood transfusions.[21] His doctoral thesis, "Banked Blood: A Study in Blood Preservation," was a landmark paper and distinguished him as an expert in blood banking.[22]

One month after Drew's return to Howard to become chairman of surgery, the news hit that the American Red Cross would no longer be accepting blood from black donors. While Drew was medical director of the Red Cross's pilot blood bank, collecting donations had always been a colorblind process.[23] When the Japanese bombed Pearl Harbor, the national blood donation program revved up and a flood of donors came forth, but black Americans were turned away. Under pressure from the NAACP, the Red Cross muted its position, and in January 1942 it announced that it would resume accepting blood from black donors but process it in different facilities and store it separately from white blood.[24]

Drew initially refrained from denouncing the segregation of blood policy, but the Red Cross's segregation of blood donations triggered something in him. He made it a point to speak out about the fact that blood donations should be classified according to individual blood types, not by race. There was no scientific basis for this discriminatory policy.

When asked if it was possible to transmit the traits and characteristics of one race to another by means of a blood transfusion, he explained that under the microscope there was no such thing as white blood or black blood. All blood looked the same. He was clinging to the hope that scientific facts would overcome prejudice, but eventually he had to give that notion up.

The blood segregation policy persisted for years. In 1944 the nation's foremost expert on blood donation, who also happened to be an African American surgeon, finally gave voice to his frustration in a speech before the NAACP: "It is with something of sorrow today that I cannot give any hope that the separation of blood will be discontinued. . . . One can say quite truthfully that on the battlefields nobody is very interested in where the plasma comes from when they are hurt. They get the first bottle they get their hands on."[25]

Drew continued to implement his vision of a tradition of excellence in surgical training at Howard University. He mentored his residents and sent the best of his trainees off to traditionally "whites only" programs such as Columbia University in New

York. Between 1941 and 1950 Drew mentored more than 50 percent of the black surgeons who became board certified.

Along the way he continued to battle the medical profession for equal rights. In 1947, Drew chided the American Medical Association (AMA) for allowing local medical societies to continue banning black physicians, thereby blocking them from membership in the national organization. He cited its "one hundred years of racial bigotry and fatuous pretense,"[26] which persisted until 1968, when the AMA finally changed its discriminatory policies at all levels so that black physicians could not be locked out of the organization.

But there was still more prejudice to overcome with his surgical colleagues. Even though Drew was chairman of an academic department of surgery, held a PhD from Columbia, was board certified and an examiner for the American Board of Surgery, and had exceeded the criteria in every way, he was not granted the rank of Fellow of the American College of Surgeons when he applied in 1945.

Drew continued pushing for equal rights, working to change the pattern of rigid desegregation of the hospitals in Washington. The only hospital where black physicians were permitted to practice was Freedmen's, even though there were black patients at other hospitals. He worked to open the doors to "white" hospitals so that black medical students, interns, and residents could train in them.[27]

Unfortunately, Drew's work was cut short by an ironic tragedy. On April 1, 1950, he was headed to a medical conference in Alabama with a group of surgeons when he fell asleep at the wheel. The car rolled several times, and Drew sustained fatal head and chest injuries. Although it was rumored for years that he was denied a life-saving blood transfusion by the segregated North Carolina hospital where he was taken, a nurse anesthetist who was monitoring Drew in the emergency room later debunked that rumor.

"We were a small hospital," she told her interviewer. "We didn't have any blood. By the time we got blood, Dr. Drew was dead."[28]

At the age of forty-four, one of America's leading surgeons, a man who had helped pioneer the nation's blood-banking system, had not been able to get the blood he so desperately needed to survive, but the accomplishments he left behind had already begun to change the course of history.

TODAY THE BLOOD SUPPLY is considered safer than it has ever been, with a chance of only 1 in 1.5 million of transmission of human immunodeficiency virus (HIV). At least a dozen tests, including hepatitis, HIV, and West Nile Virus screening, are conducted on the blood from the more than 8 million volunteers who contribute an average of 15 million units of blood in the United States.

But because human blood is still vulnerable to contamination from unpredictable future threats, a great deal of time and money has been expended trying to develop artificial blood. The military could also use a blood substitute in remote locations rather than having to rely on active-duty soldiers to donate. Patients who refuse blood transfusions for religious reasons, such as Jehovah's Witnesses, could also benefit from a blood substitute.

But just as in Charles Drew's time, when preserving blood turned out to be trickier than simply "mixing a cocktail," creating artificial blood has also turned out to be more complicated than initially imagined. Several substitutes have been tested in clinical trials, but none have managed to make it all the way to FDA approval.[29] Worrisome side effects such as elevated blood pressure, heart attacks, and strokes have impeded FDA approval.

Hemopure, a hemoglobin-based oxygen carrier produced by OPK Biotech of Cambridge, Massachusetts, is approved for use in South Africa, where the AIDS risk has been historically high. Under the FDA's compassionate care exception, six units were given to a Jehovah's Witness patient with bleeding gastrointestinal polyps in Kansas City in 2013, and no adverse effects were noted.[30]

There is another potential route to increasing the human blood supply other than donation. Blood pharming is a technique in which human red blood cells are grown from stem cells mixed with growth factors.[31] Arteriocyte, in Cleveland, Ohio, has the end goal of enabling blood to be harvested in remote areas where it is needed most, such as war zones, within the next five years.[32] If this technique proves to be commercially viable and affordable, it could avert the current infectious risks of blood donation and revolutionize the blood industry.

Whatever the source of blood in the future, we need more now than at any other point in history. Whether it is the bright crimson drained from a volunteer with a rolled-up sleeve or a straw-tinged artificial substitute concocted in a laboratory, the color of blood matters little in today's world as long as there is plenty available to fuel survival.

8 » A TOWER OF TERROR

ON AUGUST 1, 1966, ex-Marine Charles Whitman, a twenty-five-year-old architectural engineering student, introduced America to a new type of public spectacle—mass murder by firearm. From the top of the twenty-eight-story University of Texas Tower, he unleashed a torrent of bullets using a four-power scope and three rifles. He shot his first five victims inside the Tower with a sawed-off 12-gauge shotgun. A receptionist, an Air Force Academy cadet and his sixteen-year-old brother, and the boys' mother and aunt were each sprayed with pellets at close range. Three of the five would die that same day.[1]

Then the shooter climbed a flight of stairs to the observation deck of the Tower, reached into his well-stocked footlocker for a high-powered 6-millimeter Remington rifle, and aimed at eighteen-year-old Claire Wilson as she walked across campus with her boyfriend. When the pregnant coed was hit in the abdomen, the bullet went through her unborn son's skull and killed him instantly. Seconds later, Thomas Eckman, the father-to-be, slumped on top of Wilson after another missile entered his back and exploded into his chest. He too died quickly.

The severely wounded Wilson could easily have moaned, screamed, or twisted with pain, but instead she lay perfectly still.

Baking on the hot cement beneath the shield of her boyfriend's body, she was afraid to move for fear of being shot again.[2]

Whitman spent the next hour and a half picking off more victims, including a math professor headed to lunch, a Peace Corps volunteer about to leave for Iran, a high school student walking across the street, a paperboy riding his bike, a policeman who had raced to the scene, an ambulance driver loading the wounded, a reporter from the Associated Press, a merchant in a jewelry store across the street, a basketball coach in a barbershop, and an electrician who worked for the City of Austin. Anyone who moved was prey, and the expert marksman aimed to kill with each squeeze of the trigger.

Whitman attacked Austin for ninety-six minutes, across a radius of five city blocks. He took the lives of sixteen people and wounded another thirty-two.[3]

The idea that someone could be shooting people from the top of the Tower was so outside the norm of everyday life that at first observers thought the scattered bodies were the result of a fraternity prank or a play put on by the drama department. It took a few minutes for the *pop, pop, pop* to soak into people's consciousness and for them to realize that it was gunfire and they were the ones in the crosshairs.

"Random violence and mass murder wasn't something we knew. If this happened now, there would almost be a feeling of having seen it before. But we had no reference point then. We weren't even scared at first. We were just wildly curious," said Brenda Bell, who had watched the shootings from the windows of her Shakespeare class.[4]

A GUNSHOT ENTERING the body is like a miniature bomb, crushing and tearing as it spins and tumbles through organs. The bullet's path creates a trail of mangled tissue, but it also stirs up a surrounding zone of destruction that extends up to ten times the diameter of the bullet. The force stretches and shears organs, blood vessels, nerves, and muscles and compounds the damage caused by the bullet itself.

No two gunshot wounds are alike. The entrance and exit wounds might look the same from the outside, but that means almost nothing about what happened inside. The internal damage depends on a multitude of factors—bullet size, velocity, shape, spin, trajectory, distance from the gun muzzle to the target, and the position of the body as it's hit. Some bullets, meeting little in the way of resistance, travel in a straight line. Others strike a dense wall of bone and ricochet off like a pinball. Semi-jacketed hollow-point bullets mushroom on impact to increase injury.

The force of a bullet moving through the body depends on its weight and velocity.[5] The bullets fired from Whitman's 6-millimeter Remington rifle that day measured 2.82 by 0.5 inches, weighed about 6 grams (1/100th of a pound), and traveled an average of 3,500 feet per second. One well-placed shot could drop a full-sized deer from 200 yards away, more than enough firepower to kill a human.

No one was shot more than once, yet over a third of the wounded died.

Claire Wilson's one bullet was enough to rip apart her uterus, colon, stomach, and hip and kill her eight-month-old fetus. She was able to survive under a barrage of gunfire until after the shooting stopped, when she was finally transported to the operating room at Brackenridge Hospital, the first stop in a three-month stay.

Physics professor Robert Boyers's one bullet entered his lower back and shattered his kidney. He was dead on arrival.[6]

Ex-serviceman Thomas Karr's one bullet entered his left back and exited his right chest, traversing the vicinity of the ascending aorta and superior vena cava, the largest blood vessels in the body. He died on the operating room table.[7]

WHEN A SURGEON OPENS the belly of a patient with a gunshot wound, she is on a hunt, tracking the damage caused by the bullet. She doesn't know what she'll find, whether the operation will take an hour or all day, or how many units of blood will be transfused. All she knows is a patient's life is on the line and there's no other way to save them but to go in.

Her primary goal is to stop life-threatening hemorrhage, and that means she has to find the source. It is impossible to work under an opaque sea of blood and clots that obscure her view, so she must clear it all out first. To evacuate the blood she works with a combination of suction devices and sponges, packing off each region of the body cavity she's working in. This is by no means a straightforward task, and in some cases it may turn into a race against the clock.

Like a quarterback leading a hurry-up offense before halftime, she will implement her two-minute drill before time expires—that is, before the onset of profound shock that leads to death. Hopefully with this series of maneuvers, the patient's blood pressure will start to rise and approach something close to normal. But if it doesn't, or if the bleeding continues, she may have to clamp the aorta at the level of the diaphragm to try to slow down the bleeding. But even this maneuver doesn't work 100 percent of the time.

Patients still bleed to death from gunshot wounds. They bleed out at the scene. They bleed out in the ambulance. They bleed out in the operating room. And there is no mistaking that sinking feeling a first responder, nurse, or surgeon gets when the pulse fades away and the blood pressure can no longer be palpated.

In an ambulance, the next move is to start CPR. In the operating room, it is to swipe the scalpel right down the middle of the abdomen, unzip the belly, and try to hold pressure on the injury that is draining the body of blood like an oil pan without a plug. And when the abdomen opens, the organs will spill out across the drapes, soaking the towels and the floor and her shoes, but there's no going back. *What will happen next? Will the patient keep losing blood? Or will the surgeon find the holes in time and in doing so be able to reach down and pull her patient back from the edge of the cliff he toppled over?* She will know the answer shortly.

FOUR MINUTES INTO the Tower shootings, a university employee notified the Austin Police Department, but in 1966, the only possible response was to dispatch all available officers to the scene. Officer Houston McCoy was one of the first to arrive and found a campus engulfed in a sea of gunfire. Whitman was sniping from above while police and civilians who had retrieved deer rifles from home fired back at him. McCoy carried a Winchester shotgun he kept in the patrol car as he zigzagged across the campus and made his way to the Tower.

Officer Ramiro Martinez, getting dressed for work at home, turned on the TV and heard that shootings were in progress at the university campus. He too sped to the scene and made his way to the Tower equipped with only his service revolver.[8] Allen Crum, the manager of the University Co-op across the street and a twenty-two-year veteran of the U.S. Air Force, headed that way too. Crum, rifle in hand, stood guard at the door to the observation deck while Martinez and McCoy dodged civilian gunfire, subdued the sniper, and killed him.

Whitman's unprecedented actions had terrorized Austin and stunned an entire nation. President Lyndon B. Johnson ordered J. Edgar Hoover to investigate the shootings. Texas governor John Connally convened a commission of medical experts to study the shooter's behavior. The assembled panel concluded that Whitman was most likely suffering from a mental illness and that an occult brain tumor may have contributed to his actions. But there were other factors that enabled this well-executed mass murder to take place.

Whitman had seen a psychiatrist four months before the attack and articulated his mass murder vision of shooting people from the Tower with a deer rifle. But because he did not display any symptoms of "psychosis," he was steered toward outpatient therapy. No one raised a flag when he failed to appear.

Whitman purchased guns and ammunition at will in the days before the shootings. Because there was no registration requirement or a mandatory waiting period, he was able to drive from store to store assembling a large cache of murder weapons.

Everything fell into place for the shooter, and he was able to proceed without interference from anyone—not his family, his doctors, the people who sold him the guns and ammunition, or law enforcement.

IN THE AFTERMATH of the shootings, university officials closed the Tower observation deck, and for decades thereafter no memorials were erected.[9] They wanted no visual reminders of the horrific event. Bullet holes were patched on the clock face of the Tower and on buildings and sidewalks around campus.

But the law enforcement community saw an opportunity in the tragedy. They wanted to use the shootings to leverage political sentiment. Whitman's vicious assault had exposed vulnerabilities to the ever-increasing sophistication of civilian attacks. The police were at a disadvantage in apprehending heavily armed and well-positioned assailants like Whitman. Police chiefs used the Tower shootings as an impetus to form SWAT (Special Weapons and Tactics) teams trained in military Special Forces tactics and outfitted with similar gear and weapons.

In the late 1960s, after the Whitman shootings, the Los Angeles Police Department formed the nation's first SWAT team, and in 1969 they used it against the Black Panthers.[10] By 1975 there were five hundred SWAT teams in the United States, and today they number in the thousands.[11] The City of Austin formed its first SWAT team in 1979.[12]

Even smaller towns, 80 percent of those with populations ranging from twenty-five thousand to fifty thousand, have SWAT teams.

"WE HAVE ONLY two weeks, maybe only ten days before the gun lobby gets organized," President Lyndon B. Johnson (LBJ) said. "We've got to beat the NRA [National Rifle Association] into the offices of members of Congress."[13]

In 1968, the president's gun control legislation had been bottled up in the Senate Judiciary Committee for three years, and now he was looking to use the nation's outpouring of grief over the assassination of Robert F. Kennedy on June 6, 1968, to push the bill through.

At that time anyone, including minors, could walk into a store and purchase a weapon without a background check or waiting period. President John F. Kennedy's assassin had ordered his rifle through the postal service, and LBJ referred to this path as "murder by mail."

The Gun Control Act of 1968 passed only because of constant pressure on the part of the president and his aides. The bill banned all mail-order and out-of-state sales of handguns, shotguns, and rifles and prohibited the sale of guns to minors. But what infuriated LBJ was what it did *not* do: The gun lobby had killed his provision for licensing and registering guns so their use in crimes could be quickly traced back to the owner.

"We have been through a great deal of anguish these last few months and these last few years—too much anguish to forget so quickly," he said on signing the legislation.[14]

NO ONE KNEW IT at the time, but the mass shootings in Austin would mark the start of a long, still-proliferating series of mass public shootings in this country. Over the ensuing five decades, there would be ninety more mass shootings (defined as shootings in which four or more people were killed).[15] The United

States, in fact, accounts for almost a third of the world's mass shootings. Only four other countries—the Philippines (18), Russia (15), Yemen (11), and France (10)—register in the double digits for these horrific crimes.

Even more alarming is the fact that the rate of killings appears to be on the rise. After the Tower shootings in 1966, the next-highest-profile mass killing was at a McDonald's in San Ysidro, California, on July 18, 1984, when twenty-one people were killed and nineteen wounded.[16] The 1990s brought us Columbine, where two high school students killed thirteen and wounded twenty-one. The 2000s brought us Virginia Tech, where thirty-two were killed and seventeen wounded, and Fort Hood, where thirteen were killed and twenty-nine wounded.

The 2010s have been particularly disturbing, with the shooting of twenty children and six adults at Sandy Hook in 2012, the killing of twelve at the Washington Navy Yard in 2013, the killing of twenty-two people near the University of California Santa Barbara in 2014, and three more in 2015: the slaying of nine black worshippers at a church in Charleston, South Carolina; the shooting at Umpqua Community College in Roseburg, Oregon, where ten were killed and eight wounded; and a shooting and attempted bombing in San Bernardino, California, in which fourteen people were killed and twenty-two seriously injured.

And now, almost half a century later, another president's words are echoing those of the first to sign gun control legislation. During President Barack Obama's two terms in office there have been no fewer than fifteen mass shootings.[17] The president's growing sense of frustration and powerlessness in the face of a gridlocked Congress has become increasingly apparent.

"Are we really prepared to say that we're powerless in the face of such carnage, that the politics are too hard?" President Obama asked after the mass shooting at Sandy Hook Elementary School in Newtown, Connecticut, in 2012.[18]

The president vowed then to enact gun safety laws. The nation was heartbroken and the political climate seemed right, but once again gun control measures failed in 2013 in what the president described as "a shameful day" in Washington.

Nothing changed and more mass shootings followed.

"I'd ask the American people to think about how they can get our government to change these laws, and to save these lives and let these people grow up," the president said after the 2015 shootings in Oregon.

He pointed out that people have "become numb" to mass shootings and asked that an independent news organization compare the number of American deaths from terrorism versus deaths from shootings. The *Washington Post* did and found that 3,521 Americans have died from terrorist attacks since 1970, while gun violence in the country in 2015 alone has claimed 8,512.[19]

The question that begs to be answered is, Why do these gun-based mass murders keep happening in the United States? Surely we Americans are nowhere close to being as discontent as folks in the Philippines or Russia. We have a higher per capita income, better schools, greater economic opportunity, and a higher standard of living. *What is driving these shootings?*

Along with our two-car garages and 401(k)s, we have too much of something we don't need—firearms. And this, according to Adam Lankford, an associate professor of criminal justice at the University of Alabama, is at the root of the problem. "A nation's civilian firearm ownership rate is the strongest predictor of its number of mass shooters," he said.[20]

But mass shootings are not the only issue. The greater number of firearm deaths in this country occur outside these high-profile events: There are ninety single shooting deaths per day, one-third from violent crime and two-thirds from suicides.[21] Firearm casualties surround us on a day-to-day basis, but they don't get the attention that mass shootings do.

We lose an average of 100–150 people per year from mass shootings, but the loss from single-victim shootings is much greater—11,000 murders and 19,000 suicides on average, seven times higher than in the average industrial country.[22] In the year 2013, firearms killed 505 people in this country unintentionally, 11,208 intentionally, and 21,175 committed suicide. These deaths included 12 under the age of one, 39 between the ages of one and four, and 142 between the ages of five and fourteen.[23]

In the face of such alarming statistics it is easy to lose hope that anything can be done about gun violence, but Dr. Daniel Webster, director of the Johns Hopkins Center for Gun Policy and Research, believes there is hope. He predicts that over the next twenty years the United States will adopt "smarter" gun policies that will drop our murder rates by up to 30 percent.[24]

In a recent TED talk he compared the current epidemic of gun violence to the high number of motor vehicle fatalities among teenagers forty years ago. Since 1978, the number of teens killed in motor vehicle accidents has decreased by 69 percent. The dramatic drop was not achieved by banning cars or alcohol; rather, the legal standards for drunk driving were lowered, the penalties for drunk driving were raised, and merchants were held legally accountable for selling alcohol to underage drivers. Technology, such as airbags, also aided the cause.

So too, he argues, we do not need to ban guns to decrease firearm violence. We can get to that same result by enacting higher standards for gun ownership, greater accountability for those who sell guns, and better technology to keep firearms safe.

Webster's recent study from Johns Hopkins found that firearm homicides increased in Missouri when a law requiring a permit to purchase handguns ("permit-to-purchase" law) in effect since 1921 was repealed in 1997. After this change, the state murder rate from 1999 to 2012 increased by 25 percent.

The authors also looked at the effect of a Connecticut permit-to-purchase law enacted in 1995 that required a background check and an eight-hour training course before obtaining a firearm license. Firearm-related deaths dropped by 40 percent.

This data suggests that enacting higher standards for gun ownership—that is, restricting sales to those who have a criminal record or history of substance abuse—will reduce firearm-related violence. And just as those who sell alcohol to minors are held accountable, so too must we hold all gun dealers, including gun show dealers, accountable for selling guns to criminals or "straw buyers" who pass the guns along to criminals. In one example Webster describes an incident where, due to adverse publicity, a gun shop owner was held accountable for selling guns to criminals. This alone resulted in a 77 percent drop in the number of guns from that store diverted to criminals.

Advances in technology will also help deter the sale of guns to criminals. Guns can now be manufactured so that a unique microstamp is etched on any bullet fired by the gun. This microstamp would allow law enforcement to trace the bullet to the owner of the gun that fired it and identify the source of guns used in committing crimes.

New "smart gun" technology on the horizon prevents a gun from firing unless the owner is squeezing the trigger, an invaluable aid in keeping children from firing guns owned by their parents.[25] In 2015 there were forty-three instances of someone being shot by a toddler (age three or younger), resulting in thirteen deaths.[26] "Smart gun" technology would put an end to such tragedies.

The U.S. Congress might be ineffective in passing meaningful legislation, but states have been pursuing stricter gun policies in the wake of Newtown. Nearly half of all Americans now reside in states that have passed laws raising standards for gun ownership.[27] Cities are also taking action. In 2015, San Francisco passed an ordinance requiring that all gun sales be videotaped.[28]

Others are not as optimistic that gun violence will be brought under control through the passage of laws. After losing his daughter, Reema, in the 2007 Virginia Tech shootings, Joseph Samaha tried for two years to promote stiffer gun laws and ran into one roadblock after another.[29] He and other families of Virginia Tech survivors decided they weren't willing to wait around anymore and worked with public safety, mental health, and threat management experts to develop a different way to attack campus safety issues. The end result, rolled out in 2015, is the "32 National Campus Initiative," a self-assessment tool that includes nine surveys and 250 questions to help colleges and universities determine whether they have adequate safety and warning systems in place to prevent campus shootings and to make campuses safer.[30]

CLAIRE WILSON, now Claire James, returned to Austin on February 12, 2015. She came back to testify before the Texas legislature against the passage of a bill that would allow anyone twenty-one years of age and over to carry handguns on the campuses of public universities in Texas (aka "campus carry").[31]

The UT faculty council and student government had both voted to oppose campus carry. Chancellor William McRaven, a former Special Forces commander who oversaw the mission to kill Osama bin Laden, had opposed the measure as well.

But now lawmakers had a chance to hear from someone who knew firsthand what it was like to be a victim of Texas's worst mass shooting and to lose a child and a loved one in the process. "I was the first one shot in the Whitman massacre," Claire Wilson James said. "I was never able to bear children again. . . . It was a huge interruption in my young life. It's only in the last few months I've really—it's hit me how much was lost."[32]

She testified that there were so many armed civilians shooting at Whitman that rescue personnel had been unable to reach her and Thomas Eckman. Now a teacher, she urged the Senate State Affairs Committee to reject legislation that would increase the number of guns on campus.

Virginia Tech shooting victim Colin Goddard also testified. "We are not going to be able to shoot our way out of problems on college campuses," he said.[33]

Despite their testimony, and with the support of the governor, the lieutenant governor, and the overwhelming majority of lawmakers in both the House and the Senate, the bill allowing firearms to be carried on public university campuses in Texas passed.[34]

9 » OFF-ROAD MD

IT'S THE MIDDLE of the night, and Dr. Clifton Page's patient has taken a turn for the worse, with shortness of breath. Page has a treatment decision to make, but he will not be able to rely on the usual stream of data at a physician's disposal because his patient is not in an ICU, the emergency room, or a hospital room of any kind. In fact, Page can barely see or touch the patient he urgently needs to evaluate.[1]

His patient is sixty-two-year-old marathon swimmer Diana Nyad. She is treading water in the middle of the Atlantic Ocean, ten miles into an attempt at a record-breaking 110-mile swim from Cuba to Florida. Page can check Nyad's vital signs while she is in the water, but to do so would interrupt her progress while she swims over to the boat so he can press his stethoscope against her chest. Most of Page's assessment must be done by observation from a distance of six to ten feet without the benefit of labs, X-rays, or even a complete physical exam. And he must act quickly, before his patient's condition deteriorates and she has to be pulled out of the water.

AS MORE ATHLETIC ENDEAVORS are taking place off-road, outside the confines of a traditional competitive venue, medical professionals are being called upon to treat injuries and other mishaps under less than ideal conditions. The wilderness is an uncontrolled environment, subjecting athletes and adventurers to fast-moving currents, unexpected blizzards, and desiccating heat. They fall off cliffs, collapse from dehydration, and lose fingers and toes to freezing temperatures. And when they do, they may only have access to spotty medical care and few options for medical evacuation.

While the word "wilderness" conjures images of dense forests, sheer cliff faces, and raging rivers, in the realm of medical care a wilderness can crop up virtually anywhere that hospital access is farther than one to two hours away. A person could be in the wild treading water in the chilly waters off the coast of Florida, on a plateau in the Grand Canyon, inside a billowing tent at a Mount Everest base camp, or on a desolate stretch of highway shooting through West Texas. Even a city block can be transformed into a virtual wilderness by a natural disaster: In 2005 Hurricane Katrina cut people off from healthcare due to impassable streets.

Wilderness medicine is a growing field that concentrates on the treatment of patients who become injured or ill in remote or exotic locations. Its roots date back to World War II's Tenth Mountain Division, when the U.S. Army recruited eight thousand skiers and mountain climbers to fight in the Alps. Along with the ski troops came the physicians and medics to take care of them.

Dr. Albert H. Meinke Jr. served as a battalion surgeon in Italy in World War II, providing medical care at forward aid stations during the critical Riva Ridge offensive, a battle to capture contested mountain top positions in the Alps from the Germans. Because the medical team had to set up aid stations in mountainous terrain, they were forced to hike in, carrying medical supplies in rucksacks or dragging them on sleds.[2]

Evacuating the wounded from steep mountain ridges proved to be treacherous and time-consuming—each trip took up to ten hours—so army engineers devised a new method to bring them down. They stretched a cable from the top of a mountain to a valley floor so that a basket-type stretcher attached to a pulley could carry a wounded soldier to the aid station.[3] This is the kind of make-it-up-as-you-go mentality that defines wilderness medicine. Doctors are forced to innovate in the field with what few supplies they brought with them and whatever they find in nature.

After the war, the skiing soldiers and medics helped develop the National Ski Patrol, an organization founded to promote safety on the ski slope, provide instruction in winter emergency care, and rescue skiers in distress.[4] The National Ski Patrol broadened its outdoor medicine reach in the 1980s when it developed Outdoor Emergency Care, the first course directed at training emergency medical technicians to rescue the injured at ski resorts, on whitewater rafting excursions, and at other outdoor recreational settings.[5] This early outdoor medicine course covered basic life support, along with techniques for splinting extremity injuries and treating environment-induced illnesses such as heatstroke and frostbite.

Physicians from a variety of medical specialties sign on to treat injured athletes and outdoor enthusiasts, including emergency medicine physicians, trauma specialists, orthopedic surgeons, and family practice physicians specializing in sports medicine. Physicians in any specialty and medics can also take courses and become certified in Advanced Wilderness Life Support.

The demand for medical expertise to treat athletes participating in remote outdoor venues does not appear to be letting up anytime soon. Marathons and Ironman-distance triathlons, which became increasingly popular in the 1980s and '90s, are now being overshadowed by seemingly insurmountable tests of the human body and mindset in more remote locations. The greater the physical exertion and the more treacherous the terrain, the more likely medical care will be needed.

A variety of ultramarathons (distances greater than 26.2 miles) and twenty-four-hour races in which the participants run as far as they can in the time allowed now populate the fitness landscape in ever-increasing numbers and degree of difficulty. In addition to distance as a measure of exertion, terrain, weather, and even the possibility of man-made obstacles have been added to the mix, all of which increase the hazard level of a particular event and the likelihood of injury.

The Ultra-Trail du Mont Blanc, an ultramarathon that takes place in the Alps, extends 166 kilometers (103 miles) across France, Italy, and Switzerland and takes thirty to forty-five hours to complete. The Badwater, billed as the "world's toughest foot race," is a 135-mile race that starts at sea level in Death Valley and ends at Mount Whitney at an elevation of 8,360 feet. The race takes place in mid-July, when desert temperatures typically reach 120 degrees F.

Throw in the Tough Mudders, twelve-mile-long races that include fire, water, and electrical and height obstacles, and the stage is set for a host of possible mishaps. This wildly popular endurance series grew from three events in 2010 to fifty-three events globally in 2015, with ten thousand to fifteen thousand participants per event.[6]

WHEN DR. KENNETH KAMLER signed up for a mountaineering course in the 1980s, he had no idea it would lead to a new career. But then he was persuaded by his instructor to accompany a climbing expedition to Peru as the group's physician. Wilderness medicine courses hadn't yet become available; Kamler, a hand surgeon from Long Island, had to teach himself about the local threats.

Over time he developed a method for preparing for a new trip. He researched the geographic area and made a list of the possible health emergencies he might encounter, looked up the treatments, and then packed the necessary supplies in a tackle box. One such trip was to the Amazon accompanying a group of biologists studying crocodile behavior. Kamler was warned that the number-one health threat would be "getting mauled" by a crocodile, but he also prepared for the electric eel stings, piranha bites, poison frogs, and parasites that were indigenous to the area.[7]

"Humans exist within a narrow range and when people go beyond it, their bodies are not designed for it, and they may get into trouble," Kamler has said.[8]

And he should know after six trips to Mount Everest as the staff doctor for four National Geographic expeditions and two NASA-sponsored trips.[9] Everest is right up there with the most remote and difficult of medical wildernesses. Even if you bring the right supplies for every possible emergency, it is difficult to access what you need in temperatures ranging from −10 to −60 degrees F with 60-mile-an-hour winds.

But that's what Kamler did when he left his tent in one of the worst blizzards on record to try to help critically ill climbers on their way down Mount Everest in 1996. Kamler carried preloaded syringes of morphine and steroids that had frozen within minutes of stepping outside, which he thawed by sticking them under his armpit. He was forced to take some unusual steps, such as injecting patients right through their clothes rather than risk frostbite injury by peeling back their jackets to expose their skin.[10]

Kamler has a healthy respect for this most dangerous of environments and closely monitors the climbers under his medical supervision. "You really have to be careful when you go up there. People can die on a mountain. Every time I've been on Everest people have died, though not in any expedition I was a part of."[11]

At high altitude, mountaineers have low levels of oxygen in the blood, a condition known as hypoxia. The ambient barometric pressure decreases with ascending elevation, resulting in a lower partial pressure of oxygen, or "thin air." The base camp at Everest, at 17,500 feet, has a barometric pressure about half of that at sea level, and the summit has about a third.[12]

Because the body's tissues are deprived of oxygen at high altitude, climbers move much slower and can develop physiologic and neurologic problems. Throw in temperatures of an average of −4 to 10 degrees F during climbing season, and strong winds and other health problems are likely to arise, including dehydration, hypothermia, and frostbite.

"There is no rule book that says, 'When you're at 18,000 feet and this happens, do x.' Medicine freezes solid, tubing snaps in the icy winds, batteries die—nothing is predictable," said Dr. Luanne Freer, the founder of Everest ER, the mountain's only emergency care center.[13]

Kamler found that out when he sorted through the 1996 blizzard's victims, including Beck Weathers, a forty-nine-year-old pathologist from Dallas, Texas.[14]

Weathers had a dream of summiting the highest peak on each of seven continents and had two left to go when his climbing obsession took him to Nepal to summit Mount Everest in May 1996. But attempting to climb Everest, one of the most hostile and treacherous climbs, was upping the risk ante considerably.

There are a lot of ways to die on Everest: More than 240 people have been killed attempting to climb the mountain since 1953.[15] Rockslides, falling in crevasses, slipping off the edge of a cliff, being buried in an avalanche, altitude sickness, and freezing to death are the most common causes of death. Weathers's family begged him not to go, but the admitted adrenaline junkie was hooked on climbing. He assured them he'd be fine and went anyway.

Once the climb was under way, Weathers made it all the way to Camp IV or High Camp with his climbing group, led by guide Rob Hall.[16] At 25,000 feet, High Camp is located at the cusp of the Death Zone, so called because at that elevation humans develop dangerously low blood oxygen levels, and almost all require supplementary oxygen.

As the group started for the summit in the middle of the night, Weathers realized he couldn't see the face of the mountain he was walking toward. Eighteen months earlier, in an effort to improve his vision, he had undergone a radial keratotomy, an operation where small cuts are made in the cornea. What he and his ophthalmologist didn't know was that at high altitude the post-keratotomy cornea will flatten and thicken and render a person virtually blind.[17]

Weathers followed the footsteps of the person walking directly in front of him, hoping that when the sun came up his vision would improve. It did, but then he inadvertently wiped his eyes with a gloved hand and an ice crystal scratched the cornea of his right eye, leaving his vision completely blurred. Weather's guide Hall instructed him to wait until he came back and guided him down the mountain.

Weathers waited as instructed, but Hall, trapped at higher elevations in a storm, never returned; in fact, he died on the mountain. Other climbers passed Weathers on their way down and offered to help, but Weathers continued to wait. Three o'clock, the designated rendezvous time with Hall, came and went, and finally another guide and his climbers arrived on their descent. He tied Weathers to a rope and began to guide him down. By this time everyone was cold and fatigued. The descent was slow and treacherous, with intermittent slides in the ice and snow, but they were making steady progress.[18]

And then everything changed.

An hour from High Camp a monster blizzard blew in. Winds roared past at 60 miles per hour. The climbers were suddenly surrounded by dense clouds and snow, and the temperature started dropping on its way to −60. Visibility was so poor that climbers could not see the person standing next to them. Without the ability to see the next step, descending Everest was nearly impossible.

In the chaos of the incoming storm, Weathers had taken off his right outer glove and lost it. Within minutes his right hand and forearm froze solid. Conditions were so bad he couldn't even retrieve a backup glove from his backpack. The blinded Weathers was left behind with several climbers while a group left for High Camp to bring back help. At some point he became disoriented, stood up, and fell over away from the group. Some climbers were found during the storm and guided back to High Camp, but Weathers spent the night outside.

While his frostbite injuries were severe, the greatest threat to Weathers's survival in the severe cold was what was happening in his brain. Brain function is dependent on the transmission of electrical impulses between neurons, and this electrical system is very sensitive to cold. As hypothermia starts to set in and the core body temperature drops below 95 degrees F, a person becomes lethargic and confused. As body temperature continues to drop, he will develop slurred speech and may lose consciousness. Eventually a person goes into a hypothermic coma: He is completely unconscious and unresponsive to external stimuli. And at a core temperature of 68 F, brain function ceases altogether.[19]

In the extreme cold Weathers had lost consciousness and could not be aroused by a physician when he was discovered in the deep snow and ice. He was still breathing but appeared to be beyond hope. At that time on Everest no one had ever recovered from a hypothermic coma secondary to exposure. Left for dead, he lay in the snow of Everest's South Col for fifteen hours, during which time his wife in Dallas was notified that he was dead. But later that day Weathers's body warmed in the afternoon sun and he woke up.

"I looked up and the sun was above the horizon and heading down," Weathers later recalled. "So I knew that I had one more hour to live. Nobody had ever survived two nights on Everest outside."[20]

Thoughts of his wife and two children motivated him to stand up and start walking. At this point both of Weathers's hands were frozen. His cheeks and nose were blackened by frostbite. He was profoundly hypothermic, dehydrated, and nearly blind. Lacking depth perception, he struggled to make it back, falling frequently and striking his head on the ice, but he kept going and eventually found his way back to High Camp.[21] There was still little hope he would survive, but Weathers refused to die. He made it another night, drank two liters of tea, and regained some strength, and the next day, with a great deal of assistance, he made the journey from High Camp to Camp Two.

When Kamler examined Weathers and Taiwanese climber Makalu Gau at Camp Two, he discovered the worst cases of frostbite he had ever seen.[22]

"Hands, fingers, toes, all dead white, and noses, brittle black crusts," he said.[23]

Frostbite, aka cryopathy, affects body parts, particularly fingers, toes, the nose, cheeks, and ears, when they are exposed to temperatures below freezing. The degree of injury progresses and is graded similarly to a burn, from superficial frostbite, a condition where the skin blisters, turns yellow to gray, and develops a waxy feel, to deep frostbite, with an onset at 14 degrees F, where there is a greater risk of permanent damage from blood clots and gangrene.[24]

Very cold temperatures can freeze blood vessels, subcutaneous fat, muscles, and bone, and this is what happened to Beck Weathers when his right hand was left exposed and turned completely white and hard.[25] The nerves also froze, and that's why his hand was numb. Weathers's right hand could not be saved because the cold had frozen his blood vessels and stopped the circulation to his hand. The same thing happened to Weathers's nose when the skin, cartilage, and underlying bone froze.

Kamler and the medical team at base camp completely stripped Weathers, placed him in a warm sleeping bag, and started gently rewarming his hands in warm water. They infused warm intravenous fluids, drugs, and oxygen while Kamler monitored his patient as if he was in an intensive care unit. His hands were wrapped in silver nitrate bandages to keep them moist and prevent bacteria from invading the compromised tissue.

Weathers needed to get off the mountain and to a hospital, but the question was how. He'd managed to move down to Camp Two with a great deal of assistance, but he was still critically ill. The mountainous terrain would not support ground transport, and they were still forty miles from the nearest road. No helicopter had ever landed at Everest base camp because the elevation was too high and the air too thin. But Weathers's wife back in Dallas was making calls to congressmen and the state department, and as a result, she was able to arrange a helicopter rescue by Madan K. C., a Nepalese pilot.

Ultimately Weathers lost this right hand below the elbow, all the fingers of his left hand, and his nose to frostbite in this Everest disaster, which claimed the lives of eight climbers. His injuries required eleven operations, including reconstruction of his nose. He battled countless infections and unbearable physical pain. But when it was over, Weathers found himself at peace and happier than ever, his thirst for adventure finally quenched.

AFTER TWO FAILED ATTEMPTS at crossing the Florida Strait, Nyad's team learned that it is difficult to predict everything that can go wrong in the ocean. They knew they would have to deal with the hypothermia that accompanied swimming in 50-degree water for forty-eight hours and that with sleep deprivation Nyad would probably start to hallucinate. But along with the expected Nyad had also suffered a variety of unexpected ailments—a severe asthma attack, anaphylaxis from box jellyfish stings, and a shoulder injury—that added to the already Herculean task at hand.

So while preparing for the third attempt Nyad's team reached out to physicians at the University of Miami sports medicine program, and that was when Page and physician assistant Michael Letter volunteered to join the team.

At six foot four and 270 pounds, Clifton Page is as likely to be mistaken for one of the football players he treats at the University of Miami as one of the team physicians. He has had a lifelong infatuation with sports, having played tennis and basketball in high school and participated in intramural sports as an undergrad. He never fulfilled his dream of walking onto the Notre Dame basketball team, but on the way he realized another one—to become a physician: Page took a path that allowed him to stay close to the sports he loves. He went to medical school, trained in family medicine, and topped off his residency with a sports medicine fellowship to equip him to diagnose and treat athletes.

As Nyad's latest symptoms emerge, Page is getting pulled out of his sports medicine comfort zone and into territory that borders on the medically exotic. The barb-laced tentacles of the box jellyfish are lashing her body like a whip, embedding tubules into the skin of her neck, back, and arms and setting Nyad's body on fire, causing extreme pain. The tubules exude a potent neurotoxin that is not only provoking a severe allergy attack bordering on anaphylaxis but also starting to paralyze her diaphragm and nerves throughout her body.[26] Worst-case scenario: Her airway could close off from the allergic reaction. If that happened, she would no longer be able to take deep breaths or move her arms and legs.

There is no question Nyad's health is at risk, but she has invested a lot to get to this point. This is her third attempt to cross the Florida straits. Her first attempt, in 1978, was halted by bad weather after forty-two hours, more than two-thirds of the way to her goal. The second, just a year prior to this attempt, was terminated after twenty-nine hours, the combination of an eleven-hour asthma attack and a shoulder injury, sapping her of the ability to continue. The last thing Page wants to do now is to pull Nyad out of the water after she has spent the last two years, countless hours of training, and hundreds of thousands of dollars getting to this point. It is not at all certain, however, that Page will be able to deliver effective treatment while Nyad sloshes back and forth in the waves.

With a seemingly superhuman ability to block out pain, Nyad is one of the toughest patients Page has ever come across. He knows that if he can do something to improve her breathing Nyad might squeeze past this latest health crisis and complete her long-sought-after goal. On the other hand, box jellyfish stings have killed more people in the previous fifty years than shark bites, and Nyad, at sixty-two years old, is at higher risk of having an exertion-related catastrophe like a heart attack or stroke than a younger person would be.

Page is in the midst of a chilling quandary, one he has never faced before. There is no way to predict how much his patient can take before she suffers a life-threatening cardiovascular collapse or respiratory arrest, but as the senior member of the medical team, the decision is on his shoulders. What he does next will not only impact Nyad's quest to complete the 110-mile swim but could also determine whether she survives.

ONE OF THE GREATEST challenges of providing care in the wilderness is the lack of the full spectrum of equipment, instruments, and drugs used to treat patients within well-stocked hospitals. The essence of wilderness medicine is to travel light but also carry versatile tools and drugs that can play different roles depending on the emergency at hand. Physicians learn how to parlay different devices into medical tools in courses with titles like "1,001 Uses for Duct Tape and Safety Pins."[27] Safety pins alone have over twenty uses in the field, including pinning the tongue to the lower lip to establish an airway in an unconscious patient.

A basic wilderness kit is a small zippered pack stuffed with the kind of tools one doesn't usually find in a doctor's office—duct tape, safety pins, a nylon tarp, fifty feet of parachute cord, waterproof and windproof matches, adhesive foam, petroleum jelly, and a solid shank hunting knife with a six-inch blade. With a roll of duct tape, safety pins, adhesive foam, and a hunting knife, a trained wilderness medicine provider can get a good start on stabilizing just about any fracture and closing most wounds. Throw in a headlamp and they can fix them at night.

It's no wonder that Leatherman-like multitools keep showing up on lists of what to carry in a wilderness medicine kit. Carrying a multitool is like having a miniature operating room in your pocket, equipped with knife blades, scissors, a file, saw, pliers, and tweezers.

The expediency of the multitool was illustrated in 2003, when twenty-seven-year-old Aaron Ralston was pinned under an eight-hundred-pound boulder in a remote canyon in Utah. Forced to morph into his own wilderness medical team, he used a cheap multitool knockoff to amputate his arm. While the operation was anything but smooth, given the fact that the injured hiker was operating on his own body with a dull knife, Ralston performed admirably. He was still able to accomplish the task in an hour, climb out of the canyon, and hike to a nearby trail, where he was rescued.[28]

Wilderness injuries range from the frequent and mundane, like muscle strains and broken bones, to the potentially fatal, like exotic envenomations inflicted by stingrays, jellyfish, and snakes. Whatever the threat indigenous to an area, every expert agrees that being knowledgeable and prepared almost always mitigates a person's susceptibility to injury in the wild. No place is this lesson more graphically illustrated than in national parks, where spectacular scenery frequently coexists alongside the potential for grave bodily harm, separated by nothing more than a man-made barrier that beckons adventurous tourists to cross.

Every year 4.5 million people visit the Grand Canyon, and about a dozen of them die there. All told, over seven hundred people have been killed since the establishment of the canyon as a national park in 1919.[29] Visitors succumb at an average annual rate of twelve to fourteen per year.[30] One of the most common causes of avoidable death is falls, frequently linked with attempts to take or pose for a dramatic photo. All too often these misguided forays involve ignoring posted warnings and climbing over barriers and railings despite park brochures, newsletters, and signs that warn otherwise.

As reported in *Over the Edge: Death in Grand Canyon*, tragic accidents tend to follow repeatable patterns. In 1999, a twenty-five-year-old male asked nearby tourists to take his photo. He climbed over a wall and made his way to a cliff edge when he slipped on a crumbling rock and fell over nine hundred feet to his death.[31] He was not the first.

Being young and male is a "tremendous risk factor" for dying in the Grand Canyon.[32] Thirty-nine of the fifty-five people who have fallen from Grand Canyon rims were male. Other risk factors include taking what appear to be shortcuts to save time but wind up being dead ends into cliffs or worse. Hiking or climbing alone also raises the risk of accidental death or injury.[33]

While the majority of mishaps are a result of human error, some appear to be the result of bad luck. In 2012, twenty-four-year-old Ioana Hociota, a Fulbright scholar, college instructor, and seasoned climber, was hiking on a Grand Canyon trail when she stepped onto a flat ledge that gave way, dropping her down a deep chute that threw her body over a three-hundred-foot cliff edge.[34] At the time of her death she had covered over five hundred miles of the Grand Canyon and was eighty miles shy of becoming the youngest person to ever hike the entire six-hundred-mile distance. She was taking no chances and was nowhere near the cliff edge when she slipped, but in the Grand Canyon disaster can haunt even the safest path.

A year earlier in Yosemite National Park, college professor Kent Butler was hiking on the Mist Trail when he stepped aside to let other hikers pass. He slipped on a wet rock slab and was pitched into the Merced River, where he became lodged between rocks and drowned.[35] His body was retrieved a day later by a park ranger, who had to lower himself from a suspended rope into the turbulent waters to reach Butler's body.

While being the victim of a fatal fall can be categorized as being in the wrong place at the wrong time, the same cannot be said of deaths from environmental exposure, which are almost always the result of poor preparation. Summer temperatures in the Grand Canyon can reach 120 degrees during the day and continue to hover around 100 at night. The severe heat and lack of water to replenish supplies leaves hikers at risk of dehydration. Even when repeatedly advised to bring sufficient water, which may mean toting one to two gallons per person per day to stay adequately hydrated during peak temperatures, hikers frequently do not bring enough.

When a hiker runs out of water in the Grand Canyon, he still continues to lose body water from sweating and evaporation. The first symptom of dehydration is thirst, followed by a decreased urge to urinate. As the hiker continues walking for another few hours, he'll notice that his mouth is sticky and dry. He may sense his heart is racing. Thinking clearly becomes a challenge. He will feel extremely tired, and a throbbing headache may start in his temples.

As his march through the blazing canyon continues, he will become dizzy and disoriented.[36] He has just crossed the threshold from mild to moderate dehydration. Eventually his eyes will sink into the back of his head as he loses consciousness and goes into shock. He might start seizing.

If he is found at this point, he could still survive. His pulse will be rapid but thready, his breathing fast and shallow, and his blood pressure dangerously low. If he is not found within a few hours, he will most likely succumb to severe dehydration.

PAGE INITIALLY TREATS Nyad's jellyfish stings with steroid injections, Benadryl, and epinephrine.[37] At first she responds to the treatment and starts to swim again, but then she is stung again and starts to become paralyzed from the neurotoxin. In a documentary that recorded this attempt, Nyad was clearly in distress and called out, "Fire, fire," as she continued to get stung.[38]

Nyad was the only one who could terminate her arduous swim, but Page warned her that she was risking her life if she continued in the water. Reluctantly, Nyad allowed the team to pull her out of the water, and when they did so they were shocked at the welts that ringed her back and arms.

On September 2, 2013, Nyad's fifth attempt, she succeeded in swimming the 110 miles from Cuba to Florida.[39] It meant adding an anesthesiologist trained in critical care to "give Diana her best chance," Page later related. He wasn't talking about her best chance to make it across. He meant her best chance to survive if she suffered a cardiac collapse or airway emergency from anaphylaxis induced by jellyfish stings. Page deserves credit for recognizing that, as good a doctor as he is at diagnosing and treating broken bones, he would not have been the best choice for a cardiac arrest.

Nyad's team tweaked a few other key components to ensure her safety and success. Dr. Angel Yanagihara, a jellyfish expert from the University of Hawaii School of Medicine, joined the team. Dr. Yanagihara brought along an ointment she developed to neutralize the venom in jellyfish stings.[40] She jumped into the water as needed and applied the ointment when Nyad was stung.

To keep the jellyfish from stinging her lips, Nyad wore a custom silicone mask fabricated by an expert in prosthetics.[41] Nyad also wore a thin Lycra bodysuit, gloves, and booties to completely cover her skin and help keep the jellyfish at bay.[42] To counteract the effects of hypothermia Nyad drank warm broth and was showered with warm water during feedings. A navigator mapped out her route so she could swim in sync with the Gulf Stream currents.

It is hard to know whether the difference was due to the assembled expertise or the miracle of a calm-weather day, but Nyad's team had helped her overcome the wilderness of the ocean and its creatures, neutralizing as many threats as they could.

The rest had been up to her.

THREE »
POST-TRAUMA

10 » THE SAVE

HE SHUFFLED OVER, covering the hole in his neck with a shortened stub of a finger and tried to speak.

"This is me," he said, "before the fire."

It came out like a raspy whisper, barely intelligible. He pointed to a photo taped to the wall. A handsome young man in a white dress shirt, jeans, and shiny black boots looked back with a perfect smile. Then he moved to another photo of an attractive blonde and a small boy.

"My wife and son."

"Nice family," I said, nodding, doing my best to look only at the photo and not at him.

On the first day of my rotation in the burn unit in 1985, I gathered with the rest of the team to make rounds and meet the patients. The first room belonged to Jake, who'd been a roughneck on an offshore drilling rig when a pipe exploded, dousing him with flaming crude from head to toe. Within seconds he suffered third-degree burns over 98 percent of his body. Only the most protected parts, his feet and genitals, were spared. It was one of those injuries that no one is expected to survive, like a decapitation or a fall from the Empire State Building. How, all of us wondered, had he?

Jake had been flown directly from the explosion to our state-of-the-art burn center near the Texas Gulf Coast. On arrival, his neck was cut open and a tube inserted to prevent impending suffocation from smoke inhalation and swelling of his airway. During those next forty-eight hours doctors and nurses stayed parked at his bedside treating their unstable patient. They infused massive amounts of fluids into his veins that leaked into his damaged tissues. His face and everything else on him swelled to three times their normal size. When the swelling reached its peak, surgeons split the skin on his arms and legs, because they'd gotten so tight that blood couldn't flow through them.

Jake was a dead man with a beating heart if ever there was one. No one expected him to live, but there was no turning back once the battle had begun.

And over the ensuing days, powerful antibiotics and daily trips to the operating room saved him from wave after wave of invasive bacterial infections that trampled his depleted immune system and ravaged his body even more.

Jake is "quite the save," the chief resident proclaimed that day we followed him around the burn unit like chicks after a proud hen.

It was still early in my medical training, but already I had learned to dread these words. Patients like Jake, the improbable survivors of catastrophic injury, were claimed like trophies by the medical staff, but that didn't mean the price paid was worth the end result.

The last patient I met who was declared a "save" was on my psychiatry rotation. Mr. X, an untreated manic-depressive, attempted to end his life with a shotgun. As commonly happens in such scenarios, he had lost control of the long barrel, missed his brain, and splattered most of his face across the living room wall. An overachieving surgery resident flew in on the rescue helicopter, secured an airway, and brought him back to life. It was a miraculous feat but one that resulted in potentially unsolvable dilemmas.

Mr. X's head, wrapped with several brown Ace bandages, looked like a football with eyes. He could hear but could not speak. I was very green, a medical student on my psychiatry rotation, still hesitant to talk to patients and afraid to even set foot in his darkened room. *How would I communicate with him? When I looked into his eyes, would the fear I felt be reflected back?*

He held a clipboard in his hands, ready to scrawl out the answers. I looked down at my list of questions. I would never get through an exhaustive checklist of symptoms. It seemed inconsequential to probe his previous dietary habits or whether he'd suffered from migraines or skin rashes in the past. I went directly to the only question that seemed to matter.

"Yes," he wrote. He was still depressed.

Long after I left his room, thoughts of Mr. X plagued me. I was grateful that it wasn't me changing his bandages and confronting the raw hamburger lining the gaping abyss where his nose, mouth, and jaw once were. I wondered whether saving him had been the right thing to do, not just because his face was destroyed but also because he had been trying to end his life. If he was suicidal before this happened, what was he going to be like after? It would take a monumental effort to salvage what was left. Would Mr. X ever believe that this "save" had been worth the effort?

Mr. X stayed in the hospital for what seemed like years after that. Some portions of his face were reconstructed by repositioning muscle and skin from adjacent areas of his body. Other parts were fabricated out of plastic, a way to plug the holes until something better came along. Later, if you glanced at him from a distance, you might not notice a thing. Only if you got up close would you realize something was terribly wrong.

While patients can survive without a face, a severely damaged one is arguably the most socially isolating of disabilities, one invariably linked to a life-changing trauma. A face is not simply "lost," leaving behind a blank screen. It is melted away in a fire, vaporized by a shotgun, sheared off in a car wreck, or ravaged by cancer. Normal facial units—nose, mouth, eyelids, cheeks, or jawbone—are supplanted by craters, scars, or, in the worst cases, empty holes. Without a face, a person loses an identity, a mouth-piece to the world, the ability to make a living, the chance to walk down the street unnoticed.

Despite all potential obstacles—exsanguinating blood loss, overwhelming infection, airway occlusion, and simultaneous brain injury—people can and do survive. To do so entails being hospitalized for months and undergoing painful, repetitive dressing changes and numerous operations just to make it through the initial threats to life. Then begins the monumental task of restoring the intricate, one-of-a-kind, precise arrangement of skin, muscle, nerves, and cartilage by which people recognize us.

THERE IS NO MYSTERY about why the part of the body that most uniquely defines a person is so complicated to restore. The face is packed with more anatomical structures per square inch than any other region of the body. The architecture of our identities consists of twenty-four bones, each shaped to provide contour and support. There are twenty muscles on each side of the face. Eight different muscles control the tongue alone. A group of six muscles coordinate the movement of the eye ensconced in a socket formed by the delicate articulation of seven bones.

The facial nerve, which controls almost all the muscles of facial expression, has five major branches and myriad smaller ones. They fan out from just in front of each ear, the major trunks extending like fingers through the parotid gland beneath the cheek. The nose is sculpted from a combination of bone and four distinctly shaped cartilages.

THE FIRST WORLD WAR, still the benchmark for senseless carnage, resulted in an estimated 8 million dead and 21 million wounded. But there was something different about the pattern of injuries produced by this conflict. Soldiers lived and fought in an elaborate maze of trenches for months at a time, posing a new possibility of injury: If a soldier merely peered over the top, his head became the enemy's prime target. As a result, head and neck casualties were five times higher than injuries to the rest of the body, an amount and severity of facial trauma exponentially greater than at any other time in history.[1]

This virtual epidemic of facial injury was further abetted by the introduction of automatic weaponry in the early 1900s. A tripod machine gun spewed six hundred bullets per minute, any one of which could end a life or change it forever. One bullet could take out an eye with its surrounding socket, along with the forehead. One bullet could leave the jaw hanging in tatters on both sides of the lower face, gaping and raw like a newly butchered cut of meat. A single bullet might rip a nose clean off, unroof a brain, or collapse a cheek.

As maimed soldiers returned from the war in greater numbers than had ever been seen, a question emerged: What could be done to help them?

In 1914, surgery of any kind was undertaken with great caution and only as a last resort. The specialty of plastic surgery did not exist. There were no trauma centers, no intensive care units, no antibiotics, and no conceivable way to administer general anesthesia to someone without a face.

ON THE CUSP OF World War I, Harold Gillies was a young ear, nose, and throat (ENT) surgeon who had just finished his surgical training at St. Bartholomew's Hospital in London. Gillies was poised to inherit a flourishing private practice, but his plans veered off course in 1915 when he volunteered to serve with the British Red Cross in support of the war effort.[2] He was dispatched to Wimereux, France, to work with Auguste Valadier, a French American dentist who had established a dental and jaw unit in the Eighty-Third General Hospital. Trained as a dentist, Valadier was always on the verge of getting in trouble for performing surgery, and the hospital required him to operate with a medical doctor, so he conscripted Gillies as his assistant.[3]

Operating alongside Valadier, Gillies saw for the first time the devastating disfigurement that a bullet could cause and how to begin to repair the damage. Valadier, described as a rogue and a showman, had taken a radical new approach to gunshot wounds to the jaw. Rather than simply closing holes by suturing the edges together, he used tissue from other parts of the body to reconstruct unsightly defects.

Seeking more experience in head and neck surgery, Gillies next traveled to Paris to observe Europe's foremost surgeon at the time, Hippolyte Morestin. Gillies watched closely as Morestin extracted a large cancerous tumor of the face, a procedure that was not uncommon for the day. What came next, though, opened Gillies's eyes to the possibilities for reconstruction. To fill in the hole left after the tumor was removed, Morestin dissected a flap of skin from under the patient's jaw to loosen it and then rotated the flap up to fill in the surgical wound.[4]

"At that time it was the most thrilling thing I had ever seen. I fell in love with the work on the spot."[5]

Seeing this technique for the first time further cemented Gillies's interest in pursuing a field that would become known as plastic (derived from the Greek *plasticos*, meaning "fit for molding") and reconstructive surgery.[6] The specialty was virtually unknown at the time; the existing operations were performed by ENT surgeons, dentists, and general surgeons.

Treating facial injuries presented an array of challenges. Disappointing cosmetic results were inevitable, but the potential to restore a man's appearance and thus his life drew Gillies in. He headed back to England to petition the War Department to create what would become the first plastic surgery unit for the British Army. By January 1916, Gillies's efforts were rewarded with the first-time designation of a facial injury ward at the Cambridge

Military Hospital in Aldershot, the British military headquarters just outside London.

To ensure that the patients who needed his services most would be transferred to the center for the facially wounded, Gillies commissioned a stationer's shop to print labels addressed to him at the Cambridge Military Hospital. These labels were then distributed to field medics, who attached them to the uniforms of British soldiers with facial injuries. Within weeks soldiers began showing up on Gillies's doorstep, labels attached.

The newly formed facial surgery unit underwent its biggest test with the Battle of the Somme in July 1916, one of the largest and bloodiest battles of the First World War, with an estimated 1 million casualties. On the opening day alone the British army suffered fifty-eight thousand casualties, some two thousand of whom were facial trauma patients, triaged directly to Gillies. The influx swamped the resources of his fledgling ward.[7]

But rather than turn patients away, Gillies found room for every single soldier. He adroitly used the resulting cramped conditions and supply shortages to make his case for a separate hospital in which to treat the facially wounded. At his urging, the British War Department converted an old mansion in Sidcup, Kent, into a facial injury hospital that would eventually become the thousand-bed Queen's Hospital for Facial Reconstruction.

Throughout the war, soldiers poured in from the front with massive disfiguring injuries. They could barely leave the sanctuary of the hospital, much less go out in public. When severely disfigured individuals were discharged from the hospital, they were given the option of being sequestered in special housing units to avoid social ridicule. In the town of Sidcup, benches close to the hospital were painted blue, an unwritten code that indicated to passerby that men with facial disfigurement might be sitting on one.[8]

Without a face, a man's life was on hold. He couldn't mill

about in society, apply for jobs, or, in many cases, even return to his home and family. In England, severe facial disfigurement was one of the few injuries for which soldiers were granted full pensions because they were condemned to a life of social isolation.[9] The only remaining option for those who either failed repair or were not suitable candidates was to be fitted with a mask. Sculptor Anna Coleman Ladd worked out of her Studio for Portrait Masks in Paris, taking plaster casts of damaged faces and creating copper masks. She would paint each section to match the skin color of the injured man who wore it. Artist Francis Derwent Wood worked in London hospitals performing the same service.[10]

The idea for having one hospital for the facially wounded wasn't just for the purpose of housing injured soldiers but also to gather the expertise needed for complicated repairs into one location. Gillies recruited surgeons, many of whom he trained, and he also hired anesthesiologists, dentists, radiologists, and speech therapists to work together in teams. This multidisciplinary approach, now quite common in hospitals, was cutting-edge at the time. Working as part of a team fostered a synergy among the various specialties that encouraged innovation. The Queen's Hospital became by necessity both laboratory and proving ground, the site of experimentation and implementation, and out of this cauldron emerged remarkable results.[11]

Gillies chronicled his wartime reconstruction experience in a sentinel work, *Plastic Surgery of the Face: Based on Selected Cases of War Injuries of the Face Including Burns*, a virtual catalog of every conceivable facial injury that can befall a human being. The book includes chapters on repair of the cheek; injuries to the upper lip, the lower lip, and the chin; injuries of the nose, eyes, and ear; and burns to the face. Along with providing technical details and numerous photos, Gillies chronicled the personal stories of the human beings who managed to survive their injuries. Case 139 begins:

This is published, although an unfinished case. It is shown as an attempt at restoration in that not uncommon class of gunshot wound of the jaw in which the whole body of the mandible and the soft overlying tissues have been blown away en masse. It is an interesting point to note that this gallant fellow walked several miles to the dressing station on July 4th, 1916, during the Battle of the Somme, and this very feat of endurance, maintaining as he did, the upright position, may have prevented an emergency tracheostomy or even a worse fate.[12]

In the photo adjacent to the text a young man with an unshaven, swollen upper lip, short dark hair, and pale eyes stares into the camera. His tongue hangs limp, grotesquely swollen, across a ragged trail of bone and skin—all that remains of his chin and jaw.

Subsequent photos document the gradual rebuilding of the inferior third of the man's face. The lower lip reappears first. The next frame shows the tongue repositioned to the center of the mouth. Flaps harvested from the scalp and augmented with cartilage from the ribs have been transformed into a sturdy jaw. Eighteen months and six operations later, Gillies rates the outcome as satisfactory but imperfect.[13]

GILLIES FACED TWO major challenges in reconstructing facial wounds. The first was how to close complex, full-thickness injuries —the gaping holes left in the wake of a bullet. A simple skin graft could be harvested from virtually any body part and used to cover a wound, as long as there was some underlying tissue left, such as fat or muscle, to support and nourish the graft. But with gunshot wounds, that underlying tissue was frequently missing, and a graft couldn't be stretched over a hole. The second challenge was the size of the defects, some of which measured up to six inches. There simply wasn't enough spare tissue in the head and neck region to use in reconstruction. Where would the spare parts come from?

There were few existing techniques that Gillies could use on these oversized injuries. He described his work with the wounded as "a strange new art," one that he was developing one operation at a time. The stark reality of the situation was that he was regularly presented with the challenge of replacing half a face. And doing so would take more than scavenged pieces of skin, cartilage, and some horsehair suture.

The idea for a new technique came to Gillies in the operating room while he was dissecting flaps of skin and subcutaneous fat from a patient's shoulders to use in reconstruction. He noticed that the skin had a natural tendency to curl inward. He realized that if he were able to stitch opposite edges of the flaps together he could create a living tube of tissue that was still connected to its blood supply. A graft that was fed by its own blood supply was more durable and less likely to fail because it wasn't dependent on developing a new one.

Gillies called the technique of rolling skin to transfer elsewhere the tube pedicle flap. He constructed it by making two parallel incisions in a flesh-abundant region in the chest or abdomen and then rolling up the intervening patch of skin and subcutaneous fat in between them like a jellyroll.[14] Over a period of several weeks, blood vessels grew in from both ends of the tube, eventually allowing it to be disconnected from one end and transferred to an injury site.[15]

The other end of the tube remained attached to the original blood supply for several more weeks while the blood vessels grew into the tube in its newly transplanted location. Once the new blood supply was established, the other end of the tube could be safely disconnected from where it originated, the tube could be unfurled, and then it could be molded into the shape of a nose or a cheek or whatever was needed.

Within a few weeks of Gillies's discovery, flesh-colored sausages of skin began to sprout from the faces of patients awaiting reconstruction in the hospital.[16] The tube pedicle flap provided abundant extra tissue that could be molded to fit any size or shape defect, up to eight inches in length or even more when adding on an additional tube. Pulling wounds together to close a hole in the face became easier, and the inherent scars of reconstruction were minimized.

Gillies and his team performed hundreds of tube pedicle flaps on Britain's wounded soldiers. The technique was adopted worldwide, and for the next fifty years it endured as the dominant method of large-scale tissue reconstruction.

After the war, Gillies continued to work on damaged faces. Difficult cases were sent to him from surgeons worldwide—from the United States, from the rogue dentist Valadier in France, and from surgeons around the globe—with reconstructive puzzles they could not solve. Besides perfecting the tube pedicle flap, Gillies and his colleagues developed numerous facial reconstruction procedures and anesthesia techniques, many of which are still used today. Throughout his career Gillies expanded the field of reconstructive surgery to other regions of the body and became known as "the father of plastic surgery."

FAST FORWARD TO 2007, when oral and maxillofacial surgeon Colonel Robert G. Hale, assigned to Brooke Army Medical Center in San Antonio, is examining Todd Nelson's face for the first time. Nelson, a thirty-four-year-old senior logistics supervisor based in Kabul, Afghanistan, was hit by an IED that crushed his facial skeleton. His right eye and sinus cavity were ripped apart by shrapnel, and then his Toyota Land Cruiser exploded into flames that seared his face almost to the bone.[17]

Modern body armor made from ceramic plates has decreased the incidence of fatal injuries to the torso of current-day soldiers, but neither body armor nor helmets protect the face. As a result, Hale was finding that 33 to 40 percent of injured soldiers suffered facial injuries, a pattern not seen since World War I.[18]

Hale, like a modern-day Gillies, is a surgeon who inherited a menu of impossibilities and dove into finding solutions. When the reservist was deployed in 2003, first in Kuwait and later in Afghanistan, he was seeing up to fifteen patients a day with the "wicked injuries" caused by IEDs. After eleven months of active duty service he returned to his private practice briefly but then, in 2005, took the opportunity to join the teaching faculty at Brooke Army Hospital in San Antonio.

What he found was the daunting task of trying to repair damage produced by modern weaponry like IEDs with procedures that hadn't been updated for a hundred years. Hale grew frustrated with techniques that involved fashioning lips from tongues, carving out a jaw from a leg bone, and using skin, some of it too thick for the face, to cover raw wounds.

After a while he felt like he was just "dragging scar tissue around," because the end result of any operation depended on how much scar tissue developed and reclaimed his handiwork weeks after the operation.[19] Fed up with procedures that required scavenging tissue from other parts of the body and the relentless march of scar tissue, Hale went looking for other ways to deal with faces that needed rebuilding.

The first new advance he wanted to pursue was face transplant, pioneered in 2005 in France. When he approached his superiors, however, they were not enthusiastic about pursuing a solution that would require a patient to be on lifelong drugs to suppress his immune system, a necessary evil of transplanting tissue from one human to another. So Hale searched for other new technologies to improve wound healing and regenerate bone.

He worked with researchers to develop a custom-made "biomask" that can be laid over the raw surface area of a patient's burn or injury to deliver antibiotics, pump out extra fluid that causes swelling, and, in the process, minimize scarring. The biomask is now under development supported with funds from Armed Forces Institute of Regenerative Medicine (AFIRM).[20]

Hale also worked with scientists who manufacture Integra, a

skin substitute, to modify the product to be more face friendly, pliable enough to match the contours of a face. He helped develop a "spray-on skin," which can be sprayed into a raw wound to grow new cells and help close wounds faster. This product is still being tested with support from AFIRM.[21]

Meanwhile, Staff Sergeant Todd Nelson needed a face, and he couldn't wait another five years for products in the pipeline to catch up. So Hale used every procedure at his disposal to tediously reconstruct the soldier's eyelids, lips, and nose, including the use of supraclavicular flaps, a technique developed by Gillies, in which skin is harvested from the shoulders and swung up to the face to become Nelson's new cheeks.[22] Ultimately Nelson endured forty-three operations, yet the cosmetic result was, according to Hale, "far from what we'd consider normal."[23]

Eventually the military changed its mind about face transplants, even though the operation costs approximately $300,000, takes more than twenty hours to perform, and has the potential for serious lifelong complications. There are some patients who will never be able to live anything close to a normal life without a transplant, and Hale estimates there are at least two hundred veterans who would be eligible.[24]

Todd Nelson is not going to sign up for one. His face still bears the scars of his service to his country, but the basic functions necessary to live a normal life have been restored. He's had enough operations for now but continues to support any new advances that could help future victims of facial trauma.

SUBSEQUENT GENERATIONS of plastic surgeons continue to marvel at the cosmetic and functional results Gillies was able to achieve in World War I. He worked in a short-staffed hospital inundated with vast numbers of wounded and faced challenges that forced him to improvise on a daily basis. He worked on the ground floor of plastic surgery, a field that was, at the time, considered nebulous and nonessential. Yet he exceeded expectations.

It didn't matter that there were no tools or techniques, no blueprint for how to rebuild a face. It didn't matter that there were risks and failures along the way. What mattered was finding something to help the injured soldiers he treated and finding it fast. Gillies realized that if a man loses an arm or a leg he can recover and rebuild his life, but without a face, a man has little chance at getting back into the world. Gillies pushed the boundaries because restoring his patients to health required it, and as he did so he pushed the specialty of plastic surgery into existence and changed medicine forever.

11 » OUR PLASTIC BRAINS

ON JANUARY 29, 2006, newly appointed ABC news anchor Bob Woodruff was in his element, on assignment near Taji, Iraq, where he was embedded with the U.S. Fourth Infantry Division. He had only been an ABC *World News Tonight* coanchor for about a month, but like all the great ones before him, he wanted to get out on the front lines of the war and use his own words to portray the drama, not simply recite a script written by someone else.[1] And that's what he was doing, riding in the open hatch of an armored vehicle delivering a standup broadcast, when a roadside bomb exploded a mere five yards from the tank.[2]

The 155-millimeter shell that exploded, a type manufactured for cannons, measured thirty-one inches long and six inches in diameter. The Iraqi army had stockpiled hundreds of thousands of them after the Iran-Iraq War, and some were later squirreled away by insurgents after the fall of Saddam Hussein. A loaded one weighs at least a hundred pounds, depending on what kind of explosives it's packed with; the standard is a minimum of twelve pounds of TNT.

When used as IEDs, the shells are rigged with radio-controlled detonators—anything from a cellphone to a garage door opener —hidden from sight and set off remotely.[3] When the shell explodes, the steel casing breaks apart into an average of two thousand shards of metal—shrapnel—flying in all directions like an unleashed colony of bats. In the case of the bomb that hit Woodruff's armored vehicle, rocks and stones were packed around the shell to produce even more projectiles.

The concussive effect of the blast crushed Woodruff's skull over the temporal lobe of his brain, causing small spicules of bone to penetrate the underlying brain. Hundreds of pebbles and other fragments tattooed the left side of his face, his nose, and the skin around his eye. One rock sliced open his chin and fractured his jaw under the helmet line. Another, the size of a marble, shot into Woodruff's neck on the left, slipping past arteries, veins, and his trachea, and lodged one millimeter away from his right carotid artery. A larger rock threaded the armhole of his flak jacket, shattered his scapula, and left a fist-sized crater next to his chest wall.[4]

Woodruff had suffered a severe traumatic brain injury (TBI), defined as "an alteration in brain function, or other evidence of brain pathology, caused by an external force."[5] TBI has been referred to as a "signature wound" of the wars in Iraq and Afghanistan because more such injuries have been diagnosed than in any previous military conflict, an estimated 10 to 20 percent of troops, ranging from 115,000 to 350,000 soldiers.[6]

The main reasons so many are affected is the type of warfare executed in these wars—a high prevalence of IEDs, rocket-propelled grenades, and land mines—provide the ideal mechanisms to create blast injuries to the brain. Also, soldiers with severe brain injuries that might have been fatal in the past are surviving because of advances in protective gear, military medicine, and rapid air evacuation to the site of definitive care.[7]

Woodruff's brain injury was so severe that pinned to his chest was a piece of paper that read "expected," as in "expected to die."[8] At that early juncture his prospects of surviving were judged to be slim, but if he did manage to make it he would almost certainly be severely neurologically impaired.

And, just like that, in the seconds it took for an insurgent's bomb to detonate, Woodruff had changed roles from reporting the story to being the story.[9]

IT TAKES A LOT of force to break a brain, but we Americans have become experts at it. Each year in the United States approximately 1.7 million people are victims of traumatic brain injury. Of those, 1.3 million are treated and released from the emergency room, but more than 50,000 die per year, accounting for almost a third of civilian deaths from trauma.[10] Five million Americans (2 percent of the population) live with disabilities from TBI. The cost of brain injury treatment per year is estimated at more than $50 billion.

Falls, motor vehicle crashes, and assaults in which the head strikes a blunt object account for the majority of civilian head injuries. TBIS come in many different types, with a range of severity. They may be characterized as open or closed depending on whether a projectile penetrates the skull. The damage may be focused in one area, as when a particular area of the brain is bruised, or diffuse—for example, when the entire brain swells from a severe blow or a global insult such as lack of oxygen.

The Glasgow Coma Scale, a crude estimate of severity, assigns points based on eye opening, verbal response, and motor response to stimulation; scores range from 3 (severe injury with extremely poor prognosis) to 15 (mild injury with excellent prognosis). Whether a person lost consciousness and for how long (less than thirty minutes is considered mild; greater than twenty-four hours signifies severe) and the presence of amnesia are also used to classify a TBI as mild, moderate, or severe.[11]

Patients with traumatic brain injury may experience symptoms ranging from headache, memory loss, and dizziness to vomiting, lethargy, inability to move or speak, and coma.

Head trauma, like most unintentional trauma, tends to be a young person's disease. This makes it all the more tragic and costly when the victim's world is rearranged by a significant TBI that results in lifelong disability.

WOODRUFF ARRIVED by helicopter to a hospital in the Green Zone within thirty-seven minutes of the attack. From there he was flown to a forward surgical hospital in Balad. An experienced army neurosurgeon operated on him, a doctor who treated victims of explosions every single day. He opened Woodruff's skull to explore his brain and stop the bleeding. He also removed a flap of shattered bone, almost half of Woodruff's skull, and left it off, a technique known as a "decompressive craniectomy."

"We do the decompressive craniectomies . . . to counteract the swelling of the brain. . . . And since these patients sometimes have to undergo transports back to Landstuhl [Germany] and back to the States,"[12] the surgeon explained a few days later.

Military surgeons in Iraq had adopted the aggressive technique of decompressive craniectomy because the usual first-line therapy—placing a patient in a coma—requires intense continuous monitoring of a patient's brain waves and other physiologic parameters that can be difficult to carry out in the field and in transit. Woodruff's wife later commented that she was told if her husband had suffered this same injury back in the States he probably would not have survived, but because he was in the hands of surgeons who saw head wounds like his and worse every day, they knew what to do and didn't hesitate to do it.[13]

Like any body part that's been battered, a damaged brain will eventually start to swell. But unlike a broken foot, a smashed thumb, or a bruised thigh, there is only so much room inside the skull, with its three layers of unyielding bone.[14] This helmetlike structure designed to keep our fragile brains safe works against us when the brain swells beyond capacity, squeezing brain tissue and impeding cerebral blood flow. When the swelling is massive, the injured brain may start to push out of the skull anyplace it can—through a fracture if there is one, or through the base of the skull, a situation known as brain herniation, an almost uniformly fatal event.

The overall extent of brain injury is a result of a combination of the initial severity and location of the primary brain injury—the gunshot wound or brain bruise—plus the secondary effects of swelling on the brain. Because the injured brain is swollen and may have been without oxygen for some period of time, the phenomenon of secondary brain injury is in many cases a larger threat and may ultimately account for the greater degree of damage to the brain.[15] As the brain swells, the increasing pressure makes it more difficult for blood to circulate, thereby depriving the brain tissue of needed oxygen and nutrients, which in turn can cause the brain to swell more. This vicious cycle must be actively treated either with a medically induced coma or decompression to prevent the initial brain injury from being further intensified.

AS HEALERS, surgeons want to believe they can fix anything, especially when it comes to injury. How hard can it be to sew up a hole, take out an injured piece of tissue, or stop bleeding? It is an approach that works for the majority of traumatic injuries elsewhere in the body. But when it comes to the brain, neurosurgeons are working in a complicated milieu of crisscrossing neurons, each one of which has a purpose and none of which can be spared.

The sad truth is that there really is no way to repair the brain after a gunshot wound, a blow to the head, or an explosive blast. We don't know how to physically reconnect circuits that have been ripped apart by the jolt of a car crash or vaporized by high-speed projectiles. We aren't able to remove a scrambled temporal lobe and replace it with an aftermarket substitute. The most a surgeon can hope for is to find a blood clot to drain that may be putting pressure on the brain, tie off a source of bleeding, or saw out a piece of the skull to relieve pressure. What they cannot do is "fix" an injured brain or restore it to what it once was with a surgical procedure. The objective is damage control—keep the intracranial pressure as close to normal as possible, and wait to see what's left and how much of the brain will repair itself.

THE NEXT DAY, when Woodruff was stabilized after the operation, he was loaded onto a Critical Care Air Transport Team flight, essentially an intensive care unit housed within a c-17 cargo plane, a component of the Air Force Aeromedical Evacuation System. As the U.S. Air Force has reduced its in-theater medical facilities, it has developed the capabilities to rapidly evacuate even the sickest of patients to better-equipped hospitals.

Woodruff's condition was still extremely critical, but there was a limit to what could be done for him in Iraq, and more injured soldiers were rolling into the limited in-theater hospital in Balad ever day. If he was going to have the level of attention and expertise needed in a fully equipped intensive care unit he would need to be evacuated to Landstuhl Regional Medical Center in Germany, five hours away.

Picture the hollowed-out fuselage of a plane, all the seats, carpet, and plastic molding removed, so that it more closely resembles the interior of a moving van than a plane. One after another, gurneys with wounded soldiers are wheeled up the rear cargo ramp, each one surrounded by a swarm of medical personnel pushing IV poles, checking monitor screens, and inflating the lungs by hand. Each gurney will dock at an individual station outfitted with all the medical equipment and personnel available in an ICU, including one-on-one nursing, a respiratory therapist, and around-the-clock coverage from a physician trained in intensive care medicine.[16]

On arrival at Landstuhl, Woodruff was placed in a hypothermic coma to preserve brain tissue and other organs.[17] After several days he was evacuated to Bethesda Naval Hospital in Washington, D.C., where he remained in the medically induced coma for a total of thirty-six days.

REMOVING A FLAP of bone to relieve pressure in the skull after traumatic brain injury was first described in the early 1900s, but it gradually fell out of favor as modern technology and drugs developed over the last hundred years. Decompressive craniectomy, however, has made a resurgence over the last ten to fifteen years, in no small part due to the Iraq experience and war victims just like Woodruff who have benefited from the procedure. Still, the technique is considered controversial and aggressive, a last resort when all else fails to control increasing intracranial pressure. Recent clinical trials have not confirmed a clear benefit for adult TBI patients who undergo the procedure, but for children with severe head injuries, improved survival and functional improvement has been documented. Additional clinical trials are under way seeking to define this same benefit for adults.

In the meantime, in view of the many people who have undergone the procedure and emerged with "miraculous recoveries," it is hard to deny that for the right patient at the right time, removing part of the skull to relieve pressure in the brain can be a life-saving and brain-saving maneuver.

ABBY TERRELL had every reason to be enjoying life on May 26, 2015. She was exploring the Texas Hill Country with a group of friends who were visiting a cluster of wineries by bicycle. Earlier in the day she and her boyfriend had hiked up Enchanted Rock, where he had proposed on one knee and slipped a diamond and turquoise engagement ring on her finger.

By 6 p.m. the group was on the last half mile of their journey home. Abby was looking forward to calling her parents and telling them about her engagement, but she never made that call. Instead, she lost control of her bike on an unfamiliar stretch of asphalt and catapulted over the handlebars, hitting the pavement headfirst.

Local EMS responded and found her disoriented and drowsy. They placed a breathing tube, began bagging her by hand, and called for a helicopter. She was flown to the nearest trauma center, San Antonio Military Medical Center, thirty miles away. There she was admitted to the intensive care unit. Her injuries included multiple small brain bleeds (the largest was in her left temporal lobe), a hairline skull fracture, multiple facial fractures, and a shattered clavicle. Terrell's brain injury was classified as a closed head injury because there was no penetration by a projectile, but she was still very much at risk of neurologic deterioration from a swollen and bruised brain.

In the first few days after the accident her brain injury was labeled "moderate," but her brain function remained abnormal. At times she rejected medications and turned away from food except for a few sips of water. She curled up in a chair with her eyes closed, resisting attempts to engage by speech or touch. Once, while being guided to the shower, she suddenly sank to the floor, cross-legged.

Terrell's pattern of speech was described as "word salad." Even though she could pronounce words, she intermittently had difficulty finding the right ones. She had all the signs of a serious head injury—memory loss, disorientation, and difficulty speaking coherently as the day wore on—and she wasn't coming around as quickly as hoped.

After ten days in the hospital she was transferred to the Texas Institute of Rehabilitation and Research (TIRR), a rehabilitation facility closer to her home in Houston. Ranked number two in the nation by *U.S. News and World Report*, TIRR was one of the best in the country and the facility where Congresswoman Gabrielle Giffords had undergone intense rehabilitation after being shot in the head.[18]

SHORTLY AFTER Gabrielle Giffords was shot in the head from three feet away on the morning of January 8, 2011, two national news stations reported that she was dead. They were wrong, of course, but given the stark reality that 90 percent of victims of gunshot wounds to the head do not survive, the reports were all too believable. A bullet traveling at the speed of one thousand feet per second had spun through the length of her left hemisphere, shredding a six-inch core of brain. This valuable real estate controlled her speech, right-sided motor function, and immeasurable intangible qualities like charm and charisma, difficult to define, much less locate in the brain.

She too underwent a decompressive craniectomy; half of her skull was removed temporarily. According to neurosurgeons who commented on her case at the time, the pressure in her brain was relieved so quickly by the procedure that it factored into her ultimately favorable prognosis.[19]

After two weeks had passed, enough time for her egg-sized purple eyelids to return to normal, two bands of stitches to heal and to wean off the breathing machine, she opened her eyes and stared blankly at the camera her husband, Mark Kelly, used to film her progress. Unable to speak and barely able to lift two fingers on command, she was not anything close to who she had been before being shot. But what Gifford's doctors, her husband, and her therapists knew was that with aggressive rehabilitation, Gabby would get better. The question that lingered behind the optimism and enthusiasm they pushed Gabby with was, *How much better?* Gabby Giffords had been an energetic and charismatic U.S. Congresswoman who gave speeches at 270 events in one year. *How much of the old Gabby would they get back?*

HISTORICALLY, MEDICAL PROFESSIONALS were taught that our human brains had evolved to be extremely complex and that only precise areas of the brain could control specific functions. For example, the motor strip on the left side of the brain controls movement on the right side of the body, and vice versa. The ability to speak and write is controlled by the left frontal lobe (Broca's area), while a separate area in the left temporal lobe controls our ability to understand speech (Wernicke's area).[20] The right side of the brain controls creativity, spatial ability, and musical skills. The frontal lobes on both sides control our personalities, behavior, and executive functions—our ability to perform complex reasoning, make plans, and execute multistep tasks.

The downside to this conceptualization of highly specialized, irreplaceable sections was the assumption that once an area of the brain was injured, its corresponding function was irretrievably lost. According to this viewpoint, the human brain did not have the capacity to regenerate the way other organs like the liver and skin could. As a result of this ingrained teaching, physicians throughout the ages have underestimated the recovery potential of the human brain. A brain-injured patient was typically given about six weeks to demonstrate what was left, and after that they were done.

In the last several decades, however, neuroplasticity—the ability of the brain to rewire and remodel itself to compensate for loss of function in another area of the brain—began to emerge. It is believed that this happens through two mechanisms. First, the neurons immediately surrounding the injured brain cells form new connections that can bypass the injured area just like a damaged electrical circuit can be bypassed and rewired.

Second, the brain can recruit a mirror neuron in the opposite hemisphere to perform a function that can no longer be carried out in the damaged brain. In Gifford's case this would translate to recruiting the right side of the brain to control movement on the right side of the body in place of the injured left hemisphere.[21] While brain recovery can continue almost indefinitely, there is a critical period, the first three to six months after injury, when the potential for recovery is greatest. Studies have shown, however, that cognitive function can improve for at least two years after injury and possibly longer.[22]

Our understanding of brain plasticity is still unfolding. We now know not only that our brains can grow and develop in response to stimulation, but also that if we stop using a particular body part, the corresponding area of our brain will likely atrophy.[23] Dr. Norman Doidge, a leading proponent of neuroplasticity, believes that our memories and experiences are encoded in patterns of electrical energy produced by our brain cells. When a member of the string section of an orchestra is sick, a replacement can step in and play the part; similarly, a new neuron can take over for an injured one and allow the neural symphony to continue.[24]

We now know that no two brains or brain injuries are alike, that the brain can continue to repair itself for years into the future, that patients with traumatic brain injury recover better than those with brain injury caused by a stroke, and that younger patients, particularly children, may recover more function than older adults.[25]

But no one knows the limit of the brain's ability to remodel and repair itself, and for that reason alone we must err on the side of maximal rehabilitative effort for as long as a deficit remains. We must raise our expectations for recovery.

THERE COMES A TIME in the recovery process when the most serious threats to life have passed but the road ahead is still uncertain. For Bob Woodruff that time hit about mid-February 2006, about two weeks into his injury. He was in Bethesda Naval Hospital and still had not woken up. The doctors were trying to decrease his sedation, but he would get agitated and start pulling out his tubes. One day in a meeting with Bob's wife, Lee Woodruff, his neurosurgeon broached the subject of Woodruff's prognosis.

"Well, think of a baby," he said. "First they learn to speak and then to read and then to write. Bob will probably have some of these same challenges."[26]

In addition to being an accomplished broadcaster, Woodruff was a graduate of the University of Michigan Law School, fluent in French and Chinese, and the most intelligent person Lee knew.

The surgeon's statements took her aback. Until that conversation she had not contemplated a life that might include interacting with her husband as if he were a child.

She then asked if Woodruff would be able to return to work and was told he probably would not. Woodruff was so badly injured that no one knew if he would ever walk, talk, or even swallow, much less take care of himself again. And therein lies the quandary with TBI: the incredible difficulty of accurately predicting prognosis.

Despite all objective measures of injury such as the Glasgow Coma Scale (a crude measurement of prognosis based on consciousness and the ability to move the eyes and limbs) and the degree of damage seen on a CT scan of the brain, there is still no way to know how much function any individual patient will recover.

In Woodruff's case, he had defied all expectations by merely making it back to the States alive. His Glasgow Coma Scale immediately after the injury had been a 3, the lowest score possible. He had suffered a major concussive blast to the brain that caused such extensive brain swelling that his neurosurgeons in Iraq had removed half of his skull. His neurosurgeon at Bethesda had reviewed a mound of objective evidence pointing to the fact that Woodruff would have significant neurologic deficits, but even with years of experience, he had no way to know for sure.

BEFORE THE IRAQ WAR, blast injuries from IEDs or rocket-propelled grenades had not been extensively treated or understood. In addition to causing direct tissue damage to one area of the brain, such as shrapnel to the frontal lobe, blast injuries produce energy waves that are absorbed by the body. IEDs release supersonic shock waves that last only a fraction of a second but can produce pressures up to seven hundred tons traveling at up to 185 miles per hour into tissue and cause shear strain injury to organs that are not compressible, such as the brain.[27]

"It is the black box of injuries," said Dr. Alisa D. Gean, traumatic brain injury expert and chief of neuroradiology at San Francisco General Hospital.[28] Dr. Gean had observed and treated wounded soldiers at Landstuhl Regional Medical Center and admits that medical professionals are just beginning to understand them. "It is one of the most complicated injuries to one of the most complicated parts of the body."

In Iraq, soldiers were at times exposed to numerous blasts during a deployment, but escaped being diagnosed with a traumatic brain injury because they had no obvious signs of head trauma, did not lose consciousness, and continued to perform their duties.[29] A CT scan after a mild to moderate concussive injury would likely turn out normal. But later, when Iraq veterans tried to assimilate back into civilian life, they were besieged by memory loss, delayed reaction time, hearing loss, and the inability to perform executive functions that would enable them to hold down a job. They had been struck by "the invisible injury," a disorder in the brain that could not be seen from the outside and had escaped detection at the moment of impact.

When the Department of Veterans Affairs started screening Iraq and Afghanistan combat veterans, they uncovered a 15 percent incidence of previously undiagnosed mild TBI.[30] The military has become more attuned to brain injuries in returning veterans and is now performing cognitive testing before service members deploy to establish a baseline, and again when they return from deployment, as a screening tool for mild TBI.

THOSE WHO HAVE SURVIVED and even recovered most of their brain function after traumatic brain injury may be left with lasting emotional and mental consequences. Veterans of the Iraq and Afghanistan wars who suffered a traumatic brain injury have up to a 40 percent incidence of post-traumatic stress disorder (PTSD).[31] But they are also at increased risk of developing seizure disorders from brain scarring, as well as neurodegenerative disorders, including Alzheimer's disease, Lewy body dementia, and Parkinson's disease.[32] Patients who have sustained repetitive blows to the head, such as boxers and athletes who have played football, hockey, or soccer, are also at risk for chronic traumatic encephalopathy, a condition where deficits in memory, concentration, gait, and speech may develop.

IN 2011, FIVE YEARS after his traumatic brain injury, Bob Woodruff was interviewed by his former colleague Robin Roberts at ABC News about Gabrielle Giffords's injury. He had the professional appearance and cadence of any other network reporter.[33] He looked his interviewers in the eye. He gave well-thought-out answers to questions. He was animated and articulate. It was only if the camera panned from the left instead of the right that anyone could see a hint of a bulge above his left eyebrow and an indented scar near his lower jaw.

By then Woodruff had returned to broadcasting on a limited basis doing feature stories. He had also been one of the handful of critically brain injured patients who had been able to return to Bethesda Naval Hospital to shake the hands and hug the legions of healthcare workers who had helped bring him back.[34] While there he visited soldiers who were still recovering from their brain injuries. The worst of these was a young man who was in a vegetative state and unable to communicate or move.

Woodruff, moved by the plight of this soldier and of the many other injured and disabled soldiers and their families, was inspired to start a foundation that has raised more than $25 million to increase awareness of veterans' injuries and help support their recoveries. Woodruff's life had changed, but there were no indications that it was any less rewarding. He had been in a very similar situation to Gabby Giffords, and he knew the challenges she faced.

"At first you can't believe you're alive," he said, "But the recovery takes a lot longer than you ever thought."

Woodruff spoke from experience. After being in a coma for thirty-six days, he awoke with severe expressive aphasia (difficulty speaking), extensive memory loss, and generalized weakness. He required intensive physical therapy to help him learn to walk again and use his limbs, occupational therapy to help with fine motor control, speech therapy to learn to speak, and cognitive therapy to help with reasoning, judgment, and complex tasks.

As he started the rehabilitative process, he would be overcome by fatigue, alternating "good days," when he exceeded therapy expectations, with "bad days," when he was simply worn out, depressed, and unable to do much. But after forty-six days in hospitals, three weeks of inpatient rehabilitation, months of outpatient therapy, and a four-hour operation to reconstruct his skull with an acrylic plate, Bob Woodruff was able to once again take care of himself and returned to work in a profession that required perfect pitch, instant recall, charm, and superior intelligence.[35]

Knowing what he had been through and come back from when no one expected him to survive, he had high hopes for Giffords's recovery.

"If I was hit five years earlier, I really don't believe I would have survived," he later said. "I know in my heart she will recover as well."[36]

On March 15, 2015, when Lee Cowan interviewed Gabrielle Giffords and Mark Kelly for CBS Sunday Morning, Giffords looked very much like she did before the shooting.[37] She had undergone a rigorous rehabilitation process to learn how to use her still-weak right arm and leg, how to speak, and how to take care of herself again. Her husband, a former astronaut, left the space program to spend as much time as possible helping in her recovery.

She could walk, albeit with a limp, and she could speak, although finding the right words still took time. The lasting effects of her brain injury endure. She and Kelly have teamed up to form a gun control PAC and have cowritten a book, Enough, about gun violence, but she has not ruled out a return to public life.

ONE OF THE HAPPIEST days of Abby Terrell's life was the day she graduated from her TIRR rehabilitation program. It was an emotional one too. She cried tears of relief and gratitude for the love and support of her family and the dedicated staff who had helped her find her way back to the life that got put on hold in the summer of 2015.

Woodruff, Giffords, and Terrell all share membership in the TBI club. Those experiences of being transiently lost, stripped of reality, and unable to communicate will remain a part of them. All three credited the love of their families and friends with helping them find their way back to meaningful and productive lives.

For Woodruff that love got through to him even when he was in a coma. Since his injury, friends and family had been reading and talking to him waiting for a sign that Bob was still there, and for weeks they saw none.

Then one day his twelve-year-old daughter, Cathryn, whispered in his ear that she loved him.

"At that moment a tear ran down my cheek. The first sign of my return," he later wrote. "That in my opinion, is the true medicine for recovery."[38]

12 » THE TRAUMA WITHIN

OCTOBER 23, 1989. The Phillips 66 Company's Houston Chemical Complex stood as a gleaming monument to petrochemical glory at 1400 Jefferson Road near Pasadena, Texas. The plant was eight hundred acres of concrete and steel-reinforced buildings rising up to fourteen stories high, interlaced with a maze of gray pipes and beams much like an oil refinery.[1] The enormous facility could accommodate up to fourteen hundred workers at a time and produced 1.5 billion pounds a year of high-density polypropylene—white plastic pellets used to make milk bottles, produce containers, disposable razors, and toothbrushes.

A few minutes after 1 p.m., alarms in the plant began to go off. Alarms sounded all the time at the Phillips plant; most of them were mere warnings or set off by trivial malfunctions. But on this day the sound was paired with a massive vapor cloud discharging into the air from a leak in a ten-inch high-pressure pipeline carrying flammable process gas—a mixture of isobutene, ethylene, hexane, and hydrogen. The cloud immediately got the attention of workers in the vicinity. Fearing that the volatile vapor would find a spark and ignite, they scattered toward the exits, but it was too late. Within ninety seconds, eighty thousand pounds of released gas ignited and exploded with the force of 2.4 tons of TNT, strong enough to knock some workers to the ground and pitch others up into the air and fling them across the gravel.[2]

The monstrous, fuel-consuming fireball was visible from fifteen miles away. A series of secondary explosions in surrounding pipelines and storage tanks erupted like the percussion section of an orchestra. Workers were now running in all directions—anything to escape the searing heat, the dense curtain of smoke, and the hunks of metal raining down from the sky like the remnants of a doomed satellite. Within minutes the transformation from world-class chemical plant to chaotic inferno was complete.

With the plant water supply disabled by the disaster, the fire brigade could only watch in horror as the fire raged unchecked until neighboring tanker trucks responded. The extreme heat crumpled metal storage tanks the size of houses like aluminum soda cans and twisted steel beams and pipelines like straws. Search-and-rescue operations were delayed until the next morning to allow time for the scorched metal to cool.

In all, the human toll added up to 23 missing, presumed dead, and more than 130 injured, with $750 million worth of physical damage to the plant. At that time the Phillips explosion ranked as the worst industrial workplace accident since 1971, when the Occupational Safety and Health Administration had started keeping track.

Devastating injuries and economic losses were not the only damage left behind. Families of the missing waited in anguish for days for news of their loved ones: The job of identifying bodies was tediously difficult because the accident had incinerated them. The last body would not be identified until three months after the disaster.[3] Surviving workers who had literally run for their lives, climbing over walls and fences, were plagued by nightmares and anxiety.[4] Workers who still lived in the shadow of the plant feared it would erupt again. For weeks after, loud noises and sirens from neighboring plants set off waves of panic.

The day after the explosion numerous psychiatric and medical personnel arrived to assist the dazed employees and their families. The number of people who needed counseling was so large that an emergency counseling center was set up in a nearby hospital.

The most psychologically traumatized of the employees were the hundred members of the plant's fire brigade, who had responded immediately but had been largely ineffective without water. They did what they could, laying down hoses and evacuating the injured, but in doing so they had come face to face with coworkers who were moaning in agony, their clothes burned and skin charred. They saw people crushed and lacerated under heavy sheets of metal. In the ensuing days the firemen were tasked with the painful job of sorting through the debris to recover the bodies of fellow workers, some of whom they knew.

Along with family members and those involved in body recovery, three hundred employees assigned to the immediate part of the plant where the explosion started had witnessed horrific injuries and death. They too were among the emotionally devastated.

Counselors were called in to deal with the onslaught of PTSD.[5] The most common symptoms—nightmares, sleep disorders, exaggerated startle reactions, hypervigilance, and irritability—plagued the traumatized workers.[6] Emotions shifted between anxiety and fear about the future to sudden outbursts of anger at what the workers had suffered and lost. The majority had lost faith in plant management, whom they blamed for putting workers at risk, and were distrustful of the future.

Even physicians and counselors, working out of an on-site trailer, felt the effects of the trauma. The sense of tragedy shrouding the plant and the employees penetrated their professional defenses. They too were traumatized by the workers' overwhelming grief and the necessity of undertaking macabre tasks such as accompanying family members to the county morgue to identify loved ones.[7] Employees' fears about whether the plant was safe or could explode again were contagious and began to infect the counselors, who felt at a loss as to how to address the issues. They developed "compassion fatigue," a form of post-traumatic stress that affects caregivers who work long hours without an opportunity to rest and recharge.[8]

Long after the initial explosion—weeks, months, and even years later—the post-trauma shockwaves rippled through the injured survivors, the remaining workers, the families of everyone who had been present on that day, and even their caregivers.

AN ESTIMATED 7 MILLION people a year are afflicted with PTSD, a condition provoked by exposure to a traumatic event in which severe physical harm is threatened or actually occurs.[9] When it was first recognized in 1980, the traumatic event was defined as catastrophic—that is, "outside the range of normal human experience," such as occurs during war, torture, rape, a natural disaster, or an explosion like the one at the Phillips plant. Over the last several decades, however, mental health professionals began to recognize that traumatic stressors, filtered through the psychological makeup of an individual, arrive in many different packages. Even indirect exposure to the trauma, such as learning of a close friend or family member who has been raped or tortured, might evoke symptoms of PTSD.

Disasters are fertile ground for PTSD. Twenty years after the Oklahoma City bombing of 1995, in which 168 people were killed, 25 percent of survivors were found to have symptoms of PTSD.[10] In the aftermath of the 9/11 terrorist attacks on the World Trade Center, ten thousand survivors—police, firefighters, and civilians—were diagnosed with PTSD.[11] In the weeks and months after Hurricane Katrina in 2005, 38 percent of patients presenting to an emergency center were diagnosed with PTSD, ten times that of the general population.[12]

Disasters, like wars, are messy, unpredictable, and shocking. The cost exacted in human suffering seems more than we can process or understand. Yet if we or our loved ones are involved, we cannot escape the reality. The closer we are to those events, the more vivid our memories, the more continuous our playback, the more disturbed and disordered our lives can become.

The thread of PTSD symptomatology can be traced back to the Civil War, when breathless soldiers with palpitations were diagnosed with "irritable heart," a condition blamed on tight knapsack straps and strenuous marches.[13] World War I, with its trench warfare and constant barrages of heavy artillery, introduced a new name for the disorder: "shell shock," a term used to describe the mental trauma that men experienced during and after the war. World War II, in turn, came with another rebranding. This time the condition was labeled "combat exhaustion" or "battle fatigue."

No matter what name was used, little attention was paid to how to prepare a soldier to return to society afterward. Men were simply discharged and told to "go home and get to work." Initially most felt fortunate to have that opportunity after surviving wars that had inflicted so much suffering and death.[14]

By the time Vietnam vets started returning, however, it became apparent that soldiers needed help to cope—not only with the brutality of war, but also with the task of assimilating back into a society where their military service was disrespected and openly ridiculed. By 1969, a vitriolic antiwar culture had arisen, stirred by evening news reports of increasing American casualties and of atrocities committed by both sides.[15] Viewed as a quagmire, the Vietnam War was losing popular support, and American GIs were swept up in the wave of antiwar sentiment. Soldiers in uniform were openly derided as murderers and baby killers. In the years to come a rash of popular books such as *Born on the Fourth of July* and movies such as *The Deer Hunter* and *Coming Home* captured the anguish of returning Vietnam vets and suggested that even the bravest of soldiers could be trapped in the psychological web of PTSD.[16]

The military, however, refused to acknowledge that war-related

PTSD was a genuine clinical entity and would not provide treatment. Without access to the mental health services they needed, vets found other ways to get help. A grassroots movement led by the Vietnam Veterans Against the War (VVAW) sprang up and started "rap groups," meetings where soldiers could talk about the atrocities they had witnessed and taken part in.[17] Over time more vets joined, and soon the group was not only a place for informal therapy but also a strong political force with an antiwar stance.

Initially the Veterans Administration (VA) attempted to downplay the veterans' issues, but the VVAW linked up with sympathetic psychiatric professionals who gave credence and publicity to their symptoms. This prompted the Nixon administration to go on the attack against the VVAW, urging mainstream veterans organizations such as the American Legion, the Disabled American Veterans, and the Veterans of Foreign Wars to speak out against the newer group.[18]

On paper the Vietnam War ended in 1975, but the war to name the disorder that afflicted so many returning veterans continued. Without an official diagnosis sanctioned by the American Psychiatric Association (APA), it was nearly impossible to get treatment at a VA hospital. The veterans' cause was taken up by a group of psychiatrists who had supported the VVAW all along, and they continued to lobby the APA. After a series of disappointments and years of delay, post-traumatic stress disorder was finally recognized in the third edition of the *Diagnostic and Statistical Manual of Mental Disorders*, published in 1980.[19]

Soldiers would continue to come home with PTSD after the Vietnam era. Still, at least there was now a proper name for the fallout of what had happened to them mentally and emotionally while in combat. With time the U.S. Department of Veterans Affairs would fully accept and take responsibility for treating the disorder and become the home for the National Center for Post-Traumatic Stress Disorder and a leader in its treatment.[20]

Each successive conflict, including the most recent wars in Afghanistan and Iraq, demonstrated that there is no antidote to the kind of psychic and emotional trauma that can result when humans kill humans or witness violent deaths. The more frequent and intense a soldier's combat experience, the higher the risk of developing PTSD, so it is no surprise that roughly 20 percent of Iraq and Afghanistan vets are now coming home with the disorder.

One study estimated that 86 percent of soldiers in Iraq knew someone who had been killed or seriously wounded, while 68 percent reported seeing dead and wounded and 51 percent reported handling human remains.[21] The nature of counterinsurgency warfare, where attacks can come from seemingly any direction at any time, and with the possibility of civilian-initiated terrorist activities, left soldiers fearing that there was no safe place. When danger is perceived to be constant, a soldier's vigilance increases, sometimes precipitating overreaction, misplaced aggression, and increased collateral damage to civilians.

The stress of combat is worsened by the necessity for redeployments with inadequate recovery time, extensive time away from family, the disruption of civilian careers for reservists, and inadequate equipment such as armored vehicles and protective gear, which leaves soldiers vulnerable to injury and death.

VA hospitals are being overrun with PTSD patients, to the tune of approximately 476,000 per year in 2011, up from 272,000 in 2006.[22] But the patients jamming the hallways aren't just soldiers fresh from the Middle East. More than half of all new cases of PTSD are from earlier wars, including a sizable contingent of Vietnam vets who never admitted to PTSD symptoms until they retired. Without the structure of work and the pressures of raising a family to keep them busy, former soldiers had more time to reflect on their war experiences and recall traumatic events.

"It was like I had a black box on the mantel for years, but I could ignore it when I left for work every day," Vietnam vet Sam

Luna said. "When I retired, it was still sitting there, waiting for me."[23]

The VA continues to add thousands of new mental health specialists every year, but the recent epidemic of PTSD has left the military reaching for every possible solution, including groundbreaking therapies that challenge the status quo.[24]

THE POSSIBILITY OF treating patients using video game technology had first dawned on psychologist Skip Rizzo in the 1990s, when he was treating predominantly young male patients with traumatic brain injury. Rizzo made the observation that while his patients who had grown up in the digital age could be difficult to motivate during traditional talk therapy, they were eager to master video games and Nintendo 64. If he could find a way to embed therapeutic modalities in a video game, perhaps his patients would engage with these new digital tools of recovery.

At the outset of the war in Iraq, Rizzo worked at the University of Southern California–affiliated Institute for Creative Technologies, where he spent most of his day tinkering with virtual reality systems to treat attention deficit disorder in children and memory problems in adults.[25] But with the escalation of the wars in Iraq and Afghanistan, Rizzo turned his attention to adapting virtual technology to treat veterans returning with PTSD.

A major breakthrough in treating PTSD had emerged in 2000, when Dr. Edna Foa at the University of Pennsylvania developed a cutting-edge therapy known as prolonged exposure.[26] In this technique, patients are first asked to recall memories of the trauma. Then they are exposed to places and/or conditions that stimulate a more vivid recall. With time and repetition (up to twelve sessions) the stress response to the memories becomes "extinct," having been diluted by repetition. In other words, through prolonged exposure the memories lose their power.

Foa named the therapy, but veterans like Don McCarthy, a ninety-year-old former D-Day infantryman, had taken a similar approach in recovering from World War II: McCarthy visited Normandy eleven times after the war.

"If you want to get through it and live through it, and see it to its end, you gotta go back to where it was. You gotta put your feet in the water. You gotta crawl in the sand," he said. "And then you'll be all right."[27]

Rizzo researched Foa's technique and discovered other acolytes of virtual reality exposure therapy, like Dr. Barbara Rothbaum, who in 2001 had conducted a clinical study called "Virtual Vietnam," a virtual reality program to treat Vietnam vets suffering from PTSD, and Dr. JoAnn Difede, who had used virtual reality to treat survivors of the 9/11 World Trade Center attacks.

Rizzo's "aha moment" came when he discovered the video game Full Spectrum Warrior one day when he was surfing the Internet. Developed in 2000 by the Department of Defense to serve as a tactical training tool, Full Spectrum Warrior portrays actual combat maneuvers and attacks using computer animation. Rizzo's first impression was "We can use this right out of the box." And he did, initially adapting the existing game to create the first generation of Virtual Iraq, a virtual-reality-based program to simulate a typical Middle Eastern city and desert scenes where actual combat took place during the war to simulate a veteran's prior combat experience.

Today the system involves wearing sophisticated goggles and headsets with tracking devices so that as the head moves graphics rotate, making the experience even more realistic. Sounds such as engines revving, dogs barking, gunfire, and explosions are reproduced through a set of subwoofers placed under the user's chair. A smell machine emits up to eight different scents, including gunpowder, diesel fuel, burning rubber, and body odor.[28] This combination of visual, auditory, and olfactory stimuli acts together to re-create the traumatic experience that haunts a former soldier.

The system is configured so that therapists can modify the intensity of the stimuli at the same time they are monitoring the user's heart rate, breathing, and overall response to the exposure scenarios. Typically the program will begin with the user riding in a Humvee driving through the Mojave Desert stateside. As the therapy progresses, the patient narrates some of his or her experiences, and the therapist adjusts the program to simulate the terrain, weather, ambient sounds and smells, and actual events. With time and repeat exposures the narrative becomes more personal as the patient works up to re-experiencing the specific traumatizing events, such as an IED detonation that injured him or caused the death of a fellow soldier.

An early study demonstrated that approximately 80 percent of veterans benefited from virtual reality exposure therapy (VRE), many who were resistant to traditional modes of therapy.[29] A later study conducted with active-duty soldiers showed that those undergoing an average of seven sessions of VRE had significant reductions in PTSD symptoms.[30]

Exposure therapy doesn't help everyone, and some patients who have attempted it have not had good experiences. Iraq veteran David Morris underwent talk exposure therapy, without the aid of virtual reality. After a month of reliving the experience of riding in a Humvee with the sound of IEDs exploding outside, he became nauseated and stopped sleeping. He informed his counselor that the therapy was "insane and dangerous," and he quit.[31]

The success of VRE in treating PTSD prompted researchers to explore its use to prevent PTSD from developing in the first place. Rizzo and his collaborators developed STRIVE (Stress Resilience in Virtual Environments), a VRE program that exposes soldiers to traumatic events before deployment as a means of diminishing emotional reactions to stress in combat.[32] STRIVE training also builds resilience, the ability to withstand stressful situations. Soldiers are exposed to typical combat traumas, such as witnessing the death of a child or a fellow soldier. Virtual human mentors coach service members to evaluate and modify their thinking processes and behavior to produce healthier responses and develop coping skills.

The hope is that with time VRE therapy will also be adapted to treat the causes of civilian PTSD, such as traumatic accidents, rape, and abuse.

LYGIA DUNSWORTH was a registered nurse in 2003 when she underwent an operation to remove her gallbladder, normally an outpatient procedure. But she wound up developing a severe infection and pneumonia, and for months she was confined to an ICU, where she was sedated, strapped to the bed, and unable to speak because of a plastic breathing tube the size of a finger lodged in her throat.

The combination of sepsis and heavy sedation thrust her into a hallucinatory netherworld where she imagined nurses plotting to throw her into a lake, helicopters evacuating patients from a tornado, and an escape into a food freezer filled with body parts.[33] After discharge she suffered from short-term memory loss, sleep disturbances, and an irrational fear of travel, but for years she wouldn't tell anyone because of her worry that people would think she was crazy.

That same year Nancy Andrews was airlifted from Maine to Boston with a life-threatening tear in her aorta and spent two weeks in the ICU. Andrews too was subjected to heavy sedation, a breathing tube, and a tangle of tubes from IVs and EKG monitors. Looking back she was grateful for the outstanding care that saved her life but remembered the experience as a "horror" that took place in a "torture chamber."[34] She imagined being photographed by "a ring of sexual predators" who posted images on the Internet. She believed that she had hidden evidence of the crime in the sharps container on the wall and that because she was trying to stop the illicit activity, the nurses were intent on killing her. After being transferred out of the ICU and into a regular room, the sound of helicopters landing near the hospital moved Andrews to tears.

Andrews was discharged to rehab, where she learned to walk again, brush her teeth, and wash her hair, but she still feared for her safety. Once she was discharged and back at home, things didn't get a whole lot better. She couldn't tolerate even the sound of people mimicking noises that sounded like a helicopter. She burst into tears for no reason and suffered inexplicable mood swings. She wrestled with rationalizing and denying the terror she continued to feel and was afraid she would be perceived as weak and complaining.

"You tend to believe you're the only one," she said. "You wonder what is wrong with you? You made it out of the hospital, why can't you get it together?"[35]

It wasn't until she had been at home for several weeks, still seized by fear, feeling "weird," and having flashbacks, that her internist, whom she finally called, diagnosed her with PTSD over the phone.

In 2011, Sarah Wake was a recent medical school graduate training in pediatrics when she suffered a serve asthma attack while on duty at a hospital in the United Kingdom.[36] After an adverse reaction to a drug given to open her breathing passages, she was catapulted into the ICU and placed under heavy sedation. She imagined cockroaches crawling out of the eyes of an elderly patient in a bed nearby. She was convinced that blood was coming up out of cracks in her skin and overflowing onto her bed. Insects crawled up her arms and legs, and she felt smothered by the plastic mask pressed into her face. The drugs she was given to calm her anxiety, benzodiazepines, worsened her confusion and delirium, causing her to hallucinate even more vividly.

When Wake recovered and returned to work, she started a rotation in the neonatal intensive care unit, where the sounds of incessant alarms, strong odors, and disturbing sights caused her to have flashbacks of her own ICU care. She started having nightmares and dreamed of being suffocated again. One day, after a particularly busy shift, she left work and didn't return.

Even though she was a physician, Wake was unaware that the symptoms of PTSD could take weeks to months to show themselves. She was practicing active avoidance of the same stimuli she had been exposed to in the ICU—leaving her ICU rotation, taking detours to avoid the hospital, and ultimately hiding her medical textbooks—but still she did not know what was wrong.[37] She made appointments and disclosed her symptoms to her physicians but each time was "met with a blank face." No one else seemed to know what was causing her strange behavior.

Wake, like Dunsworth and Andrews, felt isolated and alone and at a loss to explain her bizarre symptoms until she started doing her own research and found other patients with similar symptoms and a name for her affliction: PTSD. After four months of psychotherapy she was able to return to work. She still has flashbacks. She still can't be around ventilators for long, but she was able to walk inside a hospital again and practice medicine.

Approximately 4.4 million patients are admitted to ICUs in the United States every year, and almost 20 percent of those surviving will develop PTSD.[38] Symptoms may persist up to six to twelve months or even longer in some patients. The fact of having a critical illness or injury alone would be traumatizing to most people, but there is something about the ICU itself that seemingly intensifies the trauma, especially for those who have a history of prior depression or anxiety.

Anyone who has been a patient in an ICU, cared for patients in one, or stayed with a hospitalized family member can relate to the experiences of these patients. The trauma of being ill is intensified by the necessities of treatment and a loss of control. ICU patients commonly have respiratory difficulties that require insertion of a breathing tube that prevents verbal communication. Patients are impaled with IVs and other monitoring devices and encumbered by wires that connect to shrill alarms. They cannot get out of bed on their own and are totally dependent on the nursing staff to help them. There is an endless cycle of pain from incisions, injuries, needlesticks, catheterizations, incessant lights, and noise and a loss of visual landmarks from awaking every day in a strange room without eyeglasses.

Patients may be strapped down to keep them from pulling out the tangle of tubes and, if showing signs of pain or anxiety, may be heavily sedated. According to one recent study, heavy and continuous sedation is a key to the formation of PTSD.[39] Sedation, while seemingly calming on the surface as a patient lapses into an unconscious state, may actually incite vivid hallucinations and nightmares. Benzodiazepines (drugs like Xanax and Valium), while administered to dampen memory and induce placidity, are some of the worst offenders when it comes to distorting reality for hospitalized patients.[40]

In the midst of the ongoing cacophony and physical insults of hospitalization, it turns out there are several simple but effective interventions. First of all, if a patient's condition allows, sedation should be periodically interrupted, giving them an opportunity to awaken from sedation and begin to establish some kind of awareness of their surroundings to assure them they are in a safe situation and not living in a continuous nightmare. Decreasing overall sedation, and particularly the use of benzodiazepines, is also a good idea.

Explaining to patients where they are and what is being done to them, especially before initiating an invasive procedure, is particularly important in decreasing the perception that they are under attack by the medical staff and the subsequent trauma that accompanies such paranoid ideations.

Keeping an ICU diary has been found to be one of the most useful tools in decreasing PTSD, as a patient can refer to it to get a sense of how long they have been in the hospital and what has occurred.[41] With conditions such as traumatic or anoxic brain injury, conditions where short-term memory may be impaired, patients frequently ask the same questions over and over: *Where am I? How did I get here? What's wrong with me?* Having an ICU journal to refer to with photos and entries by either the patient or their family members can help keep a patient on track as they review dates, familiar faces, and the progress they have made.

THE INCIDENCE OF PTSD in patients who have been the victims of traumatic injury and violent crime is greater than 20 percent, but patients at most major trauma centers are not screened for PTSD.[42] There are two reasons. First, trauma programs tend to lose money, and hospitals will not pay the extra $200,000 a year it would cost to screen trauma patients.[43] Second, even if patients are screened, there is no guarantee they would have access to mental health services after discharge, as a large percentage of trauma patients are indigent.[44] According to trauma surgeons, patients and their families remain largely uninformed about PTSD, and the lack of demand for screening and mental health services contributes to the general apathy about pursuing aggressive treatment in the trauma population.

Patients are not the only ones experiencing the wear and tear of facing near-death situations and the drastic interventions necessary to avoid them. Up to 20 percent of physicians and nurses, particularly those who work in emergency departments and intensive care units, are suffering from PTSD too.[45] Stress, repeated exposure to patients who are in severe pain with life-threatening conditions, and breaking bad news to family members are all necessary parts of the job—and can all contribute to the development of PTSD.

The emergency department (ED) in particular can be the site of confrontations and violent interactions with patients and their families.

"Almost everybody who works in the ED has been verbally assaulted by patients—every day," Dr. Leslie Zun of Mount Sinai Hospital in Chicago commented in an interview. "I'll never forget the guy who grabbed my tie and pulled me toward him and swore at me. It's a highly charged area."[46]

Specific events that can trigger a flare of PTSD include pediatric deaths, the sudden and unexpected death of a patient, medical errors, a hospital staff injury or death, a terrorist event, mass casualties, occupational needlesticks, and being sued for malpractice.[47]

One of the biggest problems medical professionals face in dealing with their own PTSD symptoms is that they are reluctant to admit to having a problem that could potentially affect their job performance, especially one that affects their mental or emotional well-being. Physicians are conditioned from early in their careers to suppress emotional responses to their patients' suffering. After years of internalizing or simply not expressing the sadness and frustrations they feel, physicians may develop severe PTSD, commonly referred to as "burnout." They are worn down mentally and physically, to the point that they cannot cope with the demands of the job and therefore simply walk away from the profession.

Emergency physician Robert Glatter believes that while most physicians learn to compartmentalize disturbing aspects of practice, many physicians have difficulty healing after traumatic on-the-job events. "The problem is that as a group, physicians don't really want to talk about it," he said.[48]

Glatter believes that emergency physicians need to take time off to recover from the traumas of the job and that meditation could be a tool to help reduce stress and anxiety.

The PTSD that physicians develop from dealing with the threat of patients dying day in and day out can also extend to caregivers of loved ones who are ill. Even months after a loved one has died, family members may have flashbacks, intrusive thoughts, and feelings of anxiety, guilt, depression, and irritability.[49]

According to Dr. Dolores Gallagher-Thompson, a psychiatrist at Stanford who has extensive experience in treating caregivers, caregiving in and of itself may not be the cause of the post-traumatic stress. Rather, a person may be at risk of PTSD because of earlier traumas in life.

After he got the call from an emergency room that his father was battling a life-threatening illness, attorney Darren Walsh wound up caring for his father full time for a year and a half. During this time Walsh found himself negotiating with hospitals and caregivers to get the best care possible for his father. "You learn whatever you thought your physical and emotional limitations were, you stretch beyond them to do what needs to be done," Walsh said.[50]

But after losing his father, Walsh found that the intensity of the memories could be overwhelming as he began to process the experience. "It's almost like your brain is careful not to open up the fire hydrant. It lets it trickle out in bits and pieces."[51]

As our population continues to age and more baby boomers move through caregiving roles and into the position of actually needing to be cared for, we are sure to learn more about the traumas of taking responsibility for a family member approaching the end of life.

TWENTY YEARS AFTER the Phillips explosion, a granite memorial inscribed with the names of the dead employees stands as a grim reminder of the loss of life and suffering that resulted from that event. But for many residents and former employees the memory of vanquished buildings and charred pipelines requires no prompting.

"I was cleaning my house trying to open my window during the explosion and it just physically threw me back," Pasadena resident Juanita Olno recalled.[52] Once the sirens started, they lasted for three days.

A former Deepwater Junior High School student remembered the explosions and sirens sounded like they came from a building next door rather than one three miles away. The school was locked down and the sirens got louder. The students had no idea what was going on.

The physical plant has long since been reconstructed, and there are few visible signs of the terror and chaos that took place on October 23, 1989, but scars remained within every human being who experienced the tragedy that day. Just like they remain in every soldier who came home from Vietnam, Iraq, and Afghanistan. Just like they remain within the ICU patients who suffered in the name of cure.

And therein lies the problem with PTSD. Bombed buildings can be rebuilt and burned skin can be excised, but what we store in our brains can never be removed.

13 » THE ROAD BACK

STAN YOO'S life-changing moment came when he was warming up on a trampoline before a gymnastics class and landed on his neck. He could move his arms, but his hands were weak and his legs wouldn't budge at all. The twenty-nine-year-old doctor was in his residency, training to become a physical medicine rehabilitation specialist. He knew immediately that he had injured his spinal cord. He also knew what would come next.[1]

Steve Shope's moment arrived in a forest near Exeter, New Hampshire, riding his mountain bike over trails he had ridden hundreds of times. The fifty-year-old geologist lost control when he scaled a four-foot-high boulder, sailed over the handlebars, and landed on his head.[2] He was being loaded into an ambulance when his wife arrived at the scene. "I'm sorry," he told her, apologizing for the accident that he knew would forever alter their lives.

On the day of their injuries, both men were thrust without warning into the ominous and uncertain world of spinal cord injury, all because of a damaged segment less than an inch or two long, the approximate length of their damaged spinal cords. Except for that one banged-up part, their bodies were otherwise intact and healthy. In fact, both amateur athletes were in excellent physical condition, but ultimately that would have little bearing on what the future held for each of them. Their fate and potential for recovery would be decided by the level at which their spines were injured and the magnitude of the disruption to the microscopic connections between one neuron and the next.[3]

AFTER A TRAUMATIC INJURY there is a flurry of intense medical activity—the rescue by first responders, a frenzied evaluation in an emergency room with life-saving procedures, trips to the operating room, days in intensive care, and possibly some near-death experiences from unexpected complications. That initial journey is filled with uncertainty, a roller-coaster ride of highs and lows, but eventually it all settles out, a steady state arrives, and out of the chaos a survivor emerges. And then another journey begins: finding the way back into the world as an independently functioning human being.

Everyone has a different path. For the majority of trauma patients this will be a short trip, nothing more than wound care instructions and a few days in physical therapy regaining muscle strength and balance. But for those who have suffered a spinal cord injury, lost limbs, been disfigured, or sustained a significant head injury, this next stage of post-trauma recovery may extend for months to years.

The rehabilitation of injury has been dubbed "the third phase of medical care," because it follows the prehospital rescue (first phase) and the acute treatment of an injury or illness (second phase). By definition, this stage of recovery is challenged by a missing body part or two or the lack of baseline motor, speech, or cognitive abilities.

A rehabilitation specialist takes whatever remains of an injured patient and makes a plan to restore as much function as possible, with the hope that even though the emerging human being won't be exactly who she was before an injury, she will one day achieve independence.

Rehabilitative specialists don't grab the headlines. You won't see them at press conferences when horrific injuries have struck.

They work behind the scenes in this under-the-radar field with a supporting cast of unsung heroes—physical, occupational, and speech therapists; cognitive psychologists, social workers, and mental health counselors—the people who shine a light on what comes next and coax a patient to come back and rejoin the world.

THE BODY IS DESIGNED to heal itself. A bone will knit its two ends back into a whole when they are held together in a plaster cast for six weeks. A torn muscle can mend in a month. The top layer of skin, sheared off by gravel or baked in the sun, will regenerate without so much as one stitch in a matter of days.

But a severed nerve will resist reuniting. It will not come back to life simply because its two ends are sewn together. Nerves regrow at a rate of about a millimeter a day from the point at which they are cut until they reach their destination.[4] Waiting for even just one nerve to grow back can be a long, tedious, and frustrating process. Some never do, and others, even if they do grow back, don't recover function.

The spinal cord is a bundle of nerves—hundreds of them. When the spinal cord sustains a significant impact that crushes, bruises or cuts it in two, the extension cord between the brain and the rest of the body has been unplugged. Surgeons usually operate immediately to take out bony fragments from fractured vertebrae that impinge on the cord and to decompress swelling. At the same time they are able to stabilize the spine with rods or plates.

After the initial injury, a second wave is triggered that extends over several days as the damage to the spinal cord extends into additional spinal segments above and below the original site of injury. High-dose steroids and therapeutic cooling of the spinal cord may help to preserve function during this acute period.[5]

Together the brain and spinal cord make up the central nervous system, the CPU of the body but they are also the most complex and unforgiving structures in the body.[6] Every millimeter of this high-dollar real estate has a function, and if even a tiny bit of it is damaged, we will notice.

From the outside the spinal cord looks like a slimy white tube. It measures about a foot and a half long and a half-inch thick, no bigger than a garter snake, but inside it is a very busy place. Motor pathways that control every movement we make share close quarters with sensory signals headed back to the brain.

There are 270,000 people living with spinal cord injury in the United States, and about 12,000 more join them each year.[7] Like trauma in general, spinal cord injury primarily affects young to middle-aged adults, 80 percent of them males. Motor vehicle crashes cause the majority, followed by falls, violence, and sports. Over 50 percent of spinal cord injuries occur at the level of the neck, the most unprotected section of the spine.

With a complete spinal cord injury, signals cannot be transmitted below the level of disruption, whether at the neck, chest, or lower back. If the cord is only stunned or partially damaged, some function will remain and hopefully more will return. But if the cord is completely disrupted, motor activity stops. Sensation disappears. Voluntary control of waste elimination is lost and sexual function is impaired. In other words, the circuit breakers have tripped. What will it take to get them up and running again?

WORKING AT A convalescent hospital where "wounded boys from the battlefield were being packed into hospitals by the planeload," Dr. Howard Rusk asked himself this question.[8] The year was 1942 and Rusk, an internist, hadn't envisioned a career working with the injured and disabled, but when the United States entered World War II, he volunteered to join the Army Air Corps and was assigned to Jefferson Barracks, a convalescent hospital in St. Louis, Missouri.

"Anyone who ever saw a planeload of them come in would never forget it—or want to see another. Boys with burns, and half their faces blown away, without arms or legs, boys with broken backs."[9]

Rusk couldn't help but notice that his patients, in various stages of recovery after combat injuries, were just lying around in their hospital beds, bored, helpless, with nothing to do. After operations and medical treatments were completed, the status quo dictated that patients be left to heal, which, in the 1940s, meant staying in bed and staring up at the ceiling. There was no coordinated plan for rehabilitating an injured soldier—no games, no talk therapy. Nothing. One soldier even complained when housekeeping came along and swept away a spider and its web above his bed because his sole source of entertainment had been swept away too.

Eventually Rusk's patients would either recover enough to be sent back to the front or be discharged to home because they were disabled. But they weren't returning home to rehabilitate, because the VA wasn't in that business. A returning soldier would have to find his own way.

Even when soldiers healed up enough to be sent back to active duty, many had no stamina and could not withstand the physical exertion of combat. A good number of the previously wounded returned to the hospital and were put back to bed, and the whole cycle started over again. As an outsider coming into the military system with fresh eyes, Rusk had a what's-wrong-with-this-picture moment.

"In the beginning, I knew only that everything possible should be done to return them to physical and mental health. This meant finding ways for them to function despite their disabilities."[10]

Rusk was not the first to make the observation that injured soldiers needed early rehabilitation. During World War I, Colonel Frank Billings had headed up a physical reconstruction division that was tasked with restoring physical and functional capabilities to wounded soldiers.[11] But in between wars the reconstruction effort shrank down to a skeleton crew. If Rusk wanted his patients to undergo active rehabilitation, he would have to reintroduce the concept to the Army Air Corps.

So Rusk, an internist with no prior experience with the disabled, designed a program of physical therapy, mental health counseling, and vocational training that included courses in practical skills like typing, accounting, and radio mechanics.

When the chief of the Air Force's medical branch heard about Rusk's program, he ordered him to Washington, D.C., to set up a convalescent training program for all 253 Air Force Hospitals.[12] Along the way Rusk met Dr. George G. Deaver, the medical director of a program for the disabled in New York who was known for getting people up and walking again. Rusk enlisted Deaver's help, and within a few weeks Rusk was sending up to two hundred physicians, therapists, and educators at a time to New York so that Deaver could train them in his techniques.[13]

The Rusk model of military rehabilitation spread from the air force to the army and, in one of his strongest legacies, was eventually adopted by the va, where it endures today.

Rusk's wartime innovations left many footprints, not the least of which was the impact of his program on spinal cord injury. According to Rusk, in World War I, four hundred soldiers became paraplegics, and 90 percent of those were dead in a year, succumbing to complications like bedsores and urinary tract infections.[14] In World War II, twenty-five hundred men became paraplegics, but 75 percent were still alive twenty years later, and over half of them were employed.[15]

After the war, Rusk had originally intended to return to his lucrative private practice in internal medicine, but over the course of the war a new dream formed—to share his wartime expertise with the world and establish the first comprehensive rehabilitation program in the United States for civilians. He approached hospitals in Missouri but could stir neither interest in nor understanding of the unknown and underappreciated field of rehabilitation medicine.

Colleagues talked about "Rusk's Folly" and labeled it a "social service boondoggle."[16] In short, friends, colleagues and family all thought he had lost his mind when he gave up the comfort and predictability of a thriving private practice for the risk and uncertainty of a new field that might never gain wide acceptance.

With the benefit of hindsight we can all nod our heads in agreement that Rusk was trying to do what made sense for the disabled. But in the 1940s and '50s the position he took was like jumping off a cliff. The disabled were hidden from view, cast aside, warehoused in cavelike institutions. No one expected them to get out of bed, much less develop into productive members of society. While the negativity gave Rusk pause, none of the criticism, not even from his own mother, was going to stop him.

Instead, he took his dream to rehabilitate the disabled to New York, where he found friendlier territory and the financial backing of financier Bernard Baruch, whom he had met during the war. Rusk was able to convince New York University (NYU) that it would be worthwhile to create a department of rehabilitation medicine.[17] New York University School of Medicine allocated two floors at Bellevue Hospital for a rehab unit for the disabled, and Rusk's program was under way.[18]

His success with the program led to his promotion to professor and chairman of the first Department of Physical Medicine and Rehabilitation at NYU. From there he established the first comprehensive training program for physicians in rehabilitation.[19] In 1950, NYU opened the Institute of Physical Medicine and Rehabilitation (later named the Howard A. Rusk Institute of Rehabilitation Medicine), the first comprehensive center devoted to care, research, and training in rehabilitation. The center's goal was to take disabled inpatients and work with them until they were able to attend schools and become employed.

But Rusk did not stop there. He continued to campaign for the rights of the disabled and "what happens to severely disabled people after the stitches are out and the fever is down," arguing that society should "take them back into the best lives they can live with what they have left."[20] He was the architect of the

"Whole Person" concept, insisting that treatment of a disabled patient not simply focus on a specific affliction, but encompass all facets of the patient's well-being, with the goal of returning that person to a role in the community.

"We had to worry about his [the patient's] emotional, social, education, and occupational needs as well. We had to treat the whole man and we had to teach his friends and his family how to accept him and help him in his new condition," Rusk said.[21]

The disabled had few advocates, much less one as vocal as Rusk, who garnered every bit of publicity he could to promote their cause, including authoring a weekly column on rehabilitation in the *New York Times* from 1946 to 1978.[22] In 1955, "Dr. Live-Again" founded the World Rehabilitation Fund to spread his philosophy around the world and start new programs to train more than six thousand physicians, psychologists, and other health specialists in over 150 countries.[23] His work continues today in Cambodia, Sierra Leone, and Afghanistan.

Rusk's body of work stretched so wide and so deep that it is difficult to believe one man could have covered so much ground. But perhaps his greatest legacy was starting a movement that transformed the care of the disabled. "To believe in rehabilitation is to believe in humanity," he wrote in his autobiography.[24] And it is obvious from his contributions that he did.

BEFORE HIS FALL on the trampoline, Stan Yoo called himself a "gym rat." A video taken before his injury proves that he could do it all—somersaults, floor exercises, elevated forward flips, artfully hoisting his body with rings. He was proud of his athleticism, and his devotion to sports had guided him to a career in rehabilitative medicine.

When he fell on November 8, 2008, he suffered a dislocation to his cervical vertebrae at the C6–C7 level in his neck. No vertebrae were broken, but his spine was unstable, and any movement would have worsened his injury. He underwent surgery within two hours of being injured, spent a week in Thomas Jefferson Hospital in Philadelphia, and then was moved to the rehab unit at Jefferson McGee. Jefferson Magee Rehabilitation Hospital is part of the Christopher and Dana Reeve Foundation's Neuro-Recovery Network, a network of cutting-edge rehabilitation centers where intensive activity-based techniques are used.[25]

Yoo knew that most of his neurologic recovery would take place in the first six months to a year after injury, and he used his insider's knowledge as motivation. "From the beginning it felt as if I was racing against the clock to get function back, and every day that I couldn't move my legs or hands was nerve-racking."

Yoo had what is known as an "incomplete" spinal cord injury: Some of his existing sensory and motor pathways were still intact. Even on the day he was injured, he could still move his arms and hands, although they were numb. When he arrived in rehab he could not move his legs, but three weeks after his injury he was able to move one leg, a sign that brain signals were getting through to his lower extremities. Shortly after that, Yoo began locomotor training, taking one step at a time with assistants on either side picking up his legs and putting them down.

The theory behind locomotor training is that even if a patient cannot yet walk, repeating the movement of walking can rebuild neural connections between the legs and the brain. He graduated to creeping up steps, concentrating on the singular act of just lifting his leg the height of a stair and then slowly setting it down.

Along the way he was able to use cutting-edge technology like a body-weight support harness that holds a person up while his legs are moved on a treadmill either by manual assistance or robotically. A physical therapist controls the input—how much load is on the patient's legs, the speed of the treadmill, and his joint angles—and provides tactile sensory cues like stroking leg tendons, while his movements simulate walking.[26]

After two months in rehab Yoo regained his ability to walk again, but that wasn't the end of the story. In one sense he was lucky—he had regained most of his function; but he still grieved the loss of his athleticism. "It's a very solitary kind of grief in that no one other than the person experiencing it will ever know just how much that person has lost. Of all the scars that can be left, I think the emotional one can quite possibly be the deepest and hardest to come back from."²⁷

STEVE SHOPE—mountain biker, surf kayaker, snowboarder, husband, and father—was also a volunteer firefighter for the Newfields Fire Department and a member of the Conservation Commission and ran his own environmental consulting company. He danced. He played the harmonica in a band and drank beer with his tight group of mountain bikers.

When he crashed his mountain bike on April 26, 2013, Steve fractured his vertebrae and damaged his spinal cord in his neck between C-5 and C-7. He suffered a "complete" spinal cord injury: He lost total motor and sensory function below the level of his injury. He underwent two operations at Beth Israel Deaconess Medical Center in Boston to stabilize and fuse his neck and then spent nine weeks at Spaulding Rehabilitation Hospital in Boston.²⁸

Almost three months later Steve returned home strapped in his wheelchair in a van. At first he was totally dependent on his wife, Julie, to feed him, dress him, and care for his other needs. Today he continues with physical therapy five days a week—two days with an exercise physiologist and five nights a week on a functional electrical stimulation (FES) bike. He has graduated from a mouth control to a joystick mounted on the arm of his wheelchair to move it. He is able to partially lift his arms and is working on feeding himself. He is back to working with his wife in their environmental engineering firm.

Steve and his wife have bills to pay—paying their kids' tuition, a mortgage, all the other financial worries of most average Americans—plus the added expense of paying for Steve's rehab equipment and all the essentials that insurance doesn't cover. They have adjusted to the new normal and gotten on with their lives.

THE LIFE EXPECTANCY of patients with spinal cord injury has improved from a lifespan measured in weeks during the 1940s to more than thirty years today.[29] Depending on the level of the injury and age at onset, most patients who survive the first year after injury can expect to live almost a normal lifespan. But despite medical advances in trauma care and intensive care medicine, the motor and sensory function of those with spinal cord injuries has refused to improve along with longevity.

Spinal cord injury victims have been waiting for decades for something new to get them up and walking, but although promising therapies are in the pipeline, to date there is no widely available "cure" for paralysis. Even in the face of the equivalent of two Manhattan Projects for spinal cord injury—the Miami Project at the University of Miami School of Medicine and the Christopher and Dana Reeve Foundation—victims of spinal cord injury have stayed in their wheelchairs.

But there is good reason to believe that things are about to change.

There are now two major directions in spinal cord research speeding toward a vast improvement in quality of life. One route is through regeneration of the spinal cord—restoring function through the use of stem cells to regrow nerves and restore connections. This approach is more complex than it sounds because of the distinct pathways running up and down the spinal cord. It is not enough to simply regenerate nerve tissue, a hard enough mission. The nerves must also find their way to the proper targets to which they were originally wired.[30]

A separate group of researchers have developed a neuro-spinal scaffold that can be inserted into the spinal cord in place of damaged tissue, which has usually liquefied or created a cystic cavity. While this therapy is still considered experimental, early results have shown improvement in motor, sensory, and bowel and bladder function, and clinical trials are ongoing.[31]

In the realm of compensating for an injury that impairs function, there is now an exoskeleton that enables a person to walk with mechanical assistance. The apparatus consists of a wearable prosthetic suit that fits from the waist down to the feet and is controlled by the user by means of a remote control worn on the wrist. For the exoskeleton to be effective, the user must have enough motor function to maneuver a set of crutches and guide the motorized movement of his legs.[32]

Dr. Miguel Nicolelis at Duke University has been working for two decades on a whole-body exoskeleton that is controlled by a brain-machine interface via an electroencephalography (EEG) cap.[33] The goal is for the electrical activity in the brain to propel the device. The suit itself includes a flexible circuit board that wraps around the extremities like a second skin through which electrical impulses are transmitted.

In the future, both repair options and compensatory devices will likely play a role in recovery from spinal cord injury depending on a patient's age and existing level of function and the presence of other disabilities or diseases.

IN NOVEMBER 2011, three years after the fall that damaged his spinal cord, a new Stanley Yoo emerged. His biceps bulged under the sleeves of his T-shirt. His shoulders had broadened. His thighs were thick and strong. The one-time gymnast, whose path had been interrupted by a stint in rehab, had morphed into a CrossFit athlete. He acknowledged that he still had deficits, that he will have them indefinitely, but you couldn't tell from the rapid cadence of his jump-roping, the way he slung a kettlebell back and forth like a piston-driven machine, or how he hoisted free weights the size of manhole covers over his head.

Yoo's journey had seemingly come full circle with one very important addition—the bottomless pit of gratitude he felt for the countless friends, family, physicians, and therapists who had helped restore him to an active life. His function had returned almost to baseline, but he was not the same man and had not forgotten where he had come from. He was still paying it forward, producing a video to thank his team while he hosted a workout fundraiser for the Christopher and Dana Reeve Foundation.[34]

While the possibility of a cure for spinal cord injury is lurking, no practical, accessible fix for complete spinal cord injury has yet arrived, and Steve Shope is not waiting around for one. He has embraced the life he has and is back to working full-time, playing the harmonica, and hanging out with his friends. He visits the bike trails he loves in a four-wheel-drive wheelchair and will soon be on a three-wheel recumbent mountain trike.

After two years of living with the highs and lows of spinal cord injury, Steve is now focused on the day-to-day realities of life just like the rest of us. But he hasn't given up on regaining the full use of his arms and legs. He is looking forward to the advances that are coming, and when someone offers him a chance to take that next step, he'll be ready.

14 » LOSING A LIMB, FINDING A CAUSE

UNLESS YOU'RE FROM Minnesota or follow the X Games, you've probably never heard of "Monster" Mike Schultz, the professional snowmobile racer who has won six gold medals at the X Games.

On December 8, 2008, Schultz was in Ironwood, Michigan, racing snocross, a sport where high-performance snowmobiles traveling at up to 60 miles per hour take on tight turns, treacherous jumps, and obstacles. Schultz, trying to come from behind, was racing down a bumpy mogul section of track in blinding snow when his snowmobile started sliding from side to side. He jumped off the machine and landed hard on his left leg with an impact too great for his knee to withstand.

He woke up with his boot lying on his chest because his leg was bent the wrong direction, a sight so unnerving that he threw the boot down where it belonged. His knee had hyperextended 180 degrees, severing his popliteal artery, vein, and nerve, behind the knee joint. When rescuers arrived and unzipped his racing leggings, blood poured out and seeped into the white snow around him.

"I knew it was bad but there was never a thought in my mind that they were going to have to amputate it."[1]

Schultz was initially taken to a small hospital in Ironwood, but it was not equipped to care for his injury. Blizzardlike conditions made helicopter evacuation impossible, so he endured a gritty two-hour ambulance ride to Duluth. Five and a half hours post-injury he was finally wheeled back to the operating room, having lost precious time when the muscles in his leg were deprived of oxygen and were slowly starting to die.

Even after the surgeon had repaired the blood vessels and blood was circulating back down to the foot, the leg just got worse. Dead tissue produced toxins that built up in his kidneys and threatened to shut them down. After the third operation the surgeons told Schultz his leg was going to have to go. He had been battling relentless pain from the moment he came down on that leg. He'd received over thirty units of blood, he was fighting infections, and nothing the doctors did was working. But he sure didn't want to lose his left leg at midthigh level. Schultz was a professional athlete at the peak of his sport, someone who made his living racing.

Game over, he thought. *Time to move onto something else.*

But to what? For him, there was nothing else. Ever since child-hood he'd been on wheels, racing three-wheelers and four-wheelers on the farm he grew up on. Wheels were an extension of his body. When he was riding and the adrenaline was surging through his veins, he came alive.

What could possibly replace that?

MORE THAN THIRTY THOUSAND arms, hands, fingers, toes, feet, and legs are crushed, pulled, or sliced off of Americans every year. The number-one cause is motorcycle or automobile crashes, followed by industrial or farm equipment. Injuries from power equipment such as electric saws, lawn mowers, and snow-blowers account for most of the rest.

When one of these patients hits the hospital, the first thing a surgeon does is make sure he is stable and has no other life-threatening injuries. Then the surgeon focuses on saving the amputated limb, either through a wholesale reattachment operation, which can take up to fifteen to twenty hours, or through a partial amputation, which involves repairing vital structures such as blood vessels and nerves.

Not every damaged extremity is a candidate for salvage. Some are too mangled to make the attempt worthwhile. If an injured limb has gone without blood flow for longer than six hours, cell death has already started to occur, and chances are the muscles and other tissues are beyond recovery. Reattachment in such cases may jeopardize the life of the patient because toxins and bacteria can flow back into the body during recirculation.

If limb viability appears borderline, surgeons will usually err on the side of keeping it, with the understanding that it may eventually have to be removed. This is what happened to Mike Schultz after three operations, when his damaged leg had begun affecting his kidneys and thus had to go.

SCHULTZ WENT THROUGH some tough times the first month after the amputation. He felt shooting pains from his leg that were so bad they felt like lightning bolts. He could still feel his foot, and there were times when he was sure he could see it.[2]

What he was going through was normal for an amputee. When someone loses a limb, it is still alive in his mind, where the neural connections that once controlled it still exist. People have clear memories of their lost limb, and they sense it too, a phenomenon known as "phantom limb." The pain associated with limb loss is from the cut nerve endings left behind in the stump. With time the sense of the limb's presence begins to fade, as does the pain, especially once a prosthetic limb is worn on a regular basis. Six weeks after the amputation, when Schultz got his first prosthesis and put weight on his leg again, his nerve pain began to subside.

People who lose a limb or other body part grieve the loss as acutely as the death of a loved one.[3] They grieve the loss of the body image they once had and perhaps even the loss of an oc-cupation that is no longer possible. In Schultz's case, he was in peak physical condition at the time of his amputation, having just spent an offseason working with a trainer and preparing for what he hoped would be a championship season. As a professional athlete, his livelihood depended on having a body that was not only intact, but could also take the day-in, day-out punishment of racing. So losing a limb didn't just change the way Schultz looked at himself in the mirror. He was sure it would change his career too.

Then he heard from another racer who was an amputee.

Jim Wazny had lost his leg in a motocross crash eight years earlier, but was back to racing when he reached out to Mike Schultz. His message was simple: With time, Schultz's pain would subside. He would walk again, run again, and, if he wanted to, even race again. The two talked on the phone, and Wazny told Schultz that the X Games also hosted adaptive competitions for disabled athletes in motocross and snowmobiles.[4]

Three months after his amputation, Schultz entered a motocross race for older racers and won. His prosthetic leg wasn't much use to him, "flopping at his side," but he was filled with hope. He was beginning to see his way to a new future. But to get there he would have to do something about that floppy leg. The problem was he couldn't find anything on the market that would provide the function he needed and still hold up to the punishment of a race.

Schultz knew nothing about making prosthetic legs, but he had built and rebuilt motorcycles and bikes for years. He could fabricate and weld metal, and knew how parts worked together. He started making sketches of how a leg built for snocross competition would work. It would have to be strong enough to absorb the energy from hundred-foot jumps in the air and also provide the flexibility and 135-degree range of motion of a human knee.

Schultz made his first prototype from cardboard and then took his design to the machine shop at Fox Racing, where he had access to all the equipment and parts he would need. Within a week the first version of the Moto Knee was born.[5] Built around a Fox compressed-air shock absorber designed for mountain bikes, the Moto Knee allows the knee joint to bend and extend like a real knee while providing a spring return on impact. Schultz attached the knee to his prosthetic foot socket when he first tried it out, and it worked just like he'd hoped. Eventually he developed the matching Versa Foot, which employs another shock absorber to enhance athletic function.[6]

Seven months after losing his leg, Schultz wore the new leg he designed in the X Games Adaptive Motocross race and won the silver medal. The next year he won the gold.

THE RECENT WARS in Iraq and Afghanistan have left a unique stamp on our military's trauma history. As in past wars, soldiers were shot, but the greater threat was explosions—roadside bombs, rocket-propelled grenades, car bombs, suicide bombers. Eighty-eight percent of wounded soldiers were blown up.[7]

Body armor and helmets offered some protection to the chest, abdomen, and brain, but extremities were still vulnerable targets. The combination of explosive devices and rapid transport to field hospitals produced an unprecedented number of soldiers surviving with more severe injuries, including amputations. Between October 7, 2001, and June 1, 2015, 1,645 soldiers, including 23 women, have suffered at least one major amputation.[8] Eighteen percent of these amputees lost more than one extremity.[9] At least 40 have lost three, and 5 have survived the loss of all four limbs.[10]

Faced with an extraordinary number of extremity injuries, the military created the Orthopedic Specialty Care Management Team to build a team of orthopedic surgeons, physical therapists, podiatrists, and occupational therapists all working together to make decisions about how best to rehabilitate amputees and salvage damaged extremities.

When an extremity has lost considerable muscle and nerves,

the function may be compromised to the point that amputation is preferable, resulting in late amputations. Fifteen percent of amputations secondary to war wounds were performed more than three months after initial injury for just this reason.[11]

Today part of the reason why a patient might choose an amputation over extensive reconstruction of a severely damaged extremity is because of the improved design and functionality of prostheses. In the last two decades prostheses have evolved from an extension that merely provides structural support and the bare minimum in function to an extremity substitute that can simulate movement and be controlled by the wearer.

Today's prosthetic legs come equipped with motorized battery-powered knees controlled by microprocessors. Their sockets are constructed of lightweight and durable carbon fiber that slip over the wearer's stump. The iWalk BiOM, a foot/ankle prosthesis that simulates the function of calf muscles and the Achilles tendon, enables the wearer to push off and move forward.[12]

Advances have also been made in hands, responsible for some of the body's most intricate and skillful movements. The iLimb Ultra is a prosthetic hand controlled by muscular movements through a myoelectric interface, giving wearers the ability to move their fingers individually and grasp objects.

As amazing as today's prostheses are, artificial limbs are on the verge of taking several significant leaps forward that will produce a more integrated responsive limb.

One of the greatest challenges facing the current generation of prostheses has been securing an artificial limb to the body. Prosthetics are dependent on having a secure, comfortable fit at the stump-socket interface, which is achieved with a cup molded to the user's stump and held into place by a strap or suction. The inherent weakness of the socket interface is that there is always soft tissue between the prosthesis and the load-bearing bone of the wearer. Stumps can get sore. They can shrink and swell, changing the fit of the prosthesis.

Researchers began studying how to integrate a prosthesis directly into the bone to avoid the soft tissue problem. They developed a new model of attachment known as "osseointegration," where an attachment rod is implanted directly into the bone. This method raised concerns about bacteria traveling from the skin-prosthesis interface and infecting the bone.

Looking to the natural world for a model, researchers examined the bond between a deer's antlers and its skull. They discovered that at the site where antlers pass through the skin they become more porous, a quality that allows the skin to grow directly into the antler, thereby closing off any route of entry for bacteria from the outside world.[13]

Researchers developed a porous titanium rod that would form the same bond between a human's prosthesis and skin as between a deer's antler and its skull. This stem is anchored into the bone during a two-stage procedure that involves first implanting a cylindrical titanium fixture directly into the bone and allowing it to heal in place for six months. The exterior portion of the rod serves as an exterior fitting that can be directly joined to a prosthesis.[14]

Mark O'Leary, a forty-year-old from London, was one of the first to receive the bone-prosthesis implant. He lauded the ease of "clicking" a prosthesis to his stump but found added benefits. "Just knowing where my foot is, my ability to know where it is improved dramatically because you can feel it through the bone," he said.[15]

The desire to feel a prosthesis, to sense how it is moving and control it with one's nerves or brain, has given rise to the field of neuroprosthetics. A neuroprosthetic is a device that supplements the input or output of the nervous system. Research is currently being conducted on neuroprostheses that substitute for limbs, the eye, general movement capability in the case of spinal cord injury, and even an implantable memory chip for the brain.

Robotic limbs controlled by human thought are already under

development. In January 2013, a truck driver in Sweden who had his arm amputated above the elbow for bone cancer had an osseo-integrated gateway, a rod with seven electrodes, implanted into his humerus.[16] After letting the gateway heal for six weeks, doctors attached a prosthetic arm to it. The implanted electrodes interact with the native nerves and muscles in the trucker's upper arm to move the prosthesis. Because the electrodes are bidirectional, they send motor impulses to the prosthesis, then relay information from the prosthesis back to the brain.

"It's very straightforward because we are using the same neural paths and muscles that were used before the amputation for prosthetic control," said Max Ortiz Catalan, one of the biomedical engineers developing the technology at the University of Technology in Gothenburg, Sweden.[17]

In a project funded by DARPA (the Defense Advanced Research Projects Agency, part of the U.S. Defense Department), researchers are creating a robotic hand with individual fingers that can perform motor functions such as picking up objects and also sense touch.[18] Increasing sensory input will improve dexterity and make the prosthesis feel more lifelike.

A 1970s television show, *The Six Million Dollar Man*, featured Colonel Steve Austin, a NASA astronaut who was severely injured when he crashed an experimental aircraft. Talented doctors rebuilt his body (both legs, one arm, and an eye) with bionic implants that enhanced his previously human function.[19] Forty years after the "six million dollar man" made his debut, we are finally on the verge of being able to create a real-life bionic man.

EVEN WITH ALL the new advances in prosthetics, the practical reality of adapting to them are still out of reach for amputees who have lost both arms. Brendan Marrocco was returning to base after a night mission at Forward Operating Base Summerall, 130 miles north of Baghdad, on April 12, 2009, when his vehicle was hit by an explosive-fired projectile. At age twenty-two, he became the first quadruple amputee from the Iraq and Afghanistan wars to survive.

Now Marrocco is the first service member to undergo a double arm transplant, performed on December 18, 2012, at Johns Hopkins University Hospital in Baltimore. His right arm was transplanted above the elbow and his left one below the elbow.

"I hated not having arms," Marrocco said after the operation. "I was all right with not having legs. Not having arms takes so much away from you."[20]

The development of limb transplantation has been delayed by ethical concerns over the lifelong need for immunosuppressive medications that can have serious side effects. Marrocco also received a bone marrow transplant in an effort to decrease the requirement for immunosuppressive medications.[21] Only six other people in the United States had undergone bilateral hand or arm transplants prior to Marrocco's.

Eighteen months after the operation Marrocco was still undergoing physical therapy but was able to push his wheelchair, stack blocks, and do pull-ups with hooks attached to his arms. His dexterity was still improving; his left hand function was significantly ahead of the right arm, which was transplanted above the elbow.[22]

It is still early in the use of hand and arm transplantation, but if these techniques prove successful over the long term, they will offer improved functionality over current upper-extremity prosthetics, which are not capable of simulating hand function and tactile abilities.

ON AUGUST 29, 2003, Keith Deutsch, a machine gunner providing rear security to a convoy, was riding in a truck struck by a rocket-propelled grenade. He sustained severe abdominal injuries, and his right leg below the knee was destroyed.[23]

Once he recovered, Deutsch, a former snowboarder, decided to take it up again. He was doing the best he could on his standard-issue prosthetic leg when he got a call from Mike Schultz. The two got together so Deutsch could try out Schultz's Moto Knee. Right away, Deutsch was able to carve in the snow, jump, and spin. Soon he was boarding just as if he had two legs again. And just like that, Schultz had his first customer.

Deutsch went on to compete in international snowboarding competitions, while Schultz formed a company, Biodapt, to produce and market the Moto Knee and Versa Foot. He's sold over two hundred, half of which are being worn by veterans who have made their way back to action sports such as motocross, snowmobiling, and competitive snowboarding.

Schultz found a natural affinity with wounded warriors from the military who, like him, wanted to rekindle the active lifestyles they had before their amputations.[24] Besides working with Deutsch, he's gotten veterans back to wakeboarding and skateboarding. He's worked with double amputees to get them snowboarding again. He's toured military bases in the Middle East and the base hospital in Germany with America 300, a group of X Games athletes. As the amputee of the group, Schultz has a special message for the other amputees he meets. *You can get in the gym again, back to lifting weights and doing CrossFit, back on your mountain bike or horse.*[25]

Mike Schultz's injury was not easy to overcome. He endured months of horrific pain and suffered the loss of a dream of competing at the highest levels as a professional athlete. But along the way to recovering he stumbled into a way to help others recover from their own life-shattering moments by doing something that plays out on a bigger stage and touches even more lives.

In losing a limb he found a cause.

DESPITE SIGNIFICANT ADVANCES in automobile safety and the success of public health initiatives like bicycle helmets and infant car seats, injury will always be with us. We will still get in car crashes, break our bones in recreational sports, and find new ways to put our bodies at risk in the outdoors. In other words, as long as we are out moving in the world, we will get hurt.

Along with the pain and suffering of being injured, we are lucky to be living in a time of sophisticated trauma care. Trained first responders come to our aid no matter where we are. Even if we are injured in a rural area, hundreds of miles from the nearest trauma center, we can be flown to one and arrive within hours of our injury. And once we are in that state-of-the-art trauma center, we will have better chances of survival than at any other time in history.

While most of us will heal from our injuries, hundreds of thousands will be burdened with a life-changing disability, such as amputation, spinal cord injury, traumatic brain injury, or the loss of vision, hearing, or an entire face. As difficult as it can be to adjust to the loss and get on with life, the good news is that with recent scientific advances people can make their way back from many disabilities, and that number will only expand in the future.

We can already transplant a missing hand. One day we may be able to regrow one in the laboratory. We are on the verge of being able to replace an extremity with an incorporated bionic arm or leg; we may soon be able to do the same for the brain with implantable memory chips. Spinal cord injury can already improve through novel and intensive therapies such as locomotor training, but in the future we will be able to repair that two-inch gap in the power cord of life.

But first we must survive the initial injury.

And thanks to the work of many dedicated individuals spread across decades of discovery, most of us will.

ACKNOWLEDGMENTS

In every war from the Civil War through the current day, our wounded troops and their physicians, nurses, and medics made numerous sacrifices. The field of trauma medicine was born out of those sacrifices, and this new area of expertise has carried over to our civilian population and made our lives safer.

My agent, Laurie Abkemeier, is a constant source of guidance and helped shape the story of trauma medicine into a book. My editor, Stephen Hull, made this journey with me through wars and hospitals and all their detours and provided much-needed direction. I was extremely fortunate to again work with the talented and insightful Christi Stanforth as my copyeditor.

Hurt is filled with stories of heroes—survivors of trauma and their families, surgeons, helicopter pilots, soldiers, and scientists. I wish to thank Dr. Randall Holland, Katie Holland, and Dr. Hugh Foy for providing information about Katie's inspiring story of survival. Dr. Clifton Page shared his expertise as a sports medicine physician. I am grateful to Abby Terrell for sharing her personal experience as a trauma patient.

Sue Baker, the "queen of public health," provided details of her pioneering work. Military historian Mat Moten read parts of the manuscript for accuracy. My brother Chris Musemeche consulted on firearm capability. Steve and Julie Shope, the epitome of courage and grace, shared insights into living with spinal cord injury.

Spike Gillespie read parts of the manuscript, asked all the right questions, and spurred me to the finish. My research assistant Taylor Yarborough hunted down references with fervor. The University of Texas Libraries and their friendly and cooperative staff were an outstanding resource. I am especially grateful to my first reader, Anne Morgan, who edited with her keen eye for detail and grammar and provided unending support.

NOTES

1. ALONG FOR THE RIDE

1. National Academy of Sciences, *Accidental Death and Disability: The Neglected Disease of Modern Society* (Washington, DC: National Academy of Sciences, 1966), www.ems.gov/pdf/1997-reproduction -accidentaldeathdissability.pdf.

2. "Historical Highlights: The Highway Safety Act of 1966," http:// history.hous.gov/Historical-Highlights/1951-2000/The-Highway-Safety -Act-of-1966, accessed January 6, 2015.

3. Lyndon B. Johnson, "Remarks at the Signing of the National Traffic and Motor Vehicle Safety Act and the Highways Safety Act," September 9, 1966, posted at *The American Presidency Project*, ed. John T. Woolley and Gerhard Peters, www.presidency.ucsb.edu/ws/?pid=27847.

4. James K. Styner, "Guest Editorial: The Birth of Advanced Trauma Life Support," *Journal of Trauma Nursing* 13 (2006): 41–44, www.nursingcenter .com/journalarticle?article_ID=655757.

5. American College of Surgeons Committee on Trauma (ACS-COT), *Advanced Trauma Life Support for Doctors: ATLS Student Course Manual*, 8th ed. (Chicago: ACS-COT, 2008), xx.

6. "Advanced Life Support: The Past to the Present," *Resuscitation Council Newsletter*, Suppl. (Summer 2011): https://www.resus.org.uk /_resources/assets/attachment/full/0/1997.pdf. See also Styner, "Guest Editorial: The Birth of Advanced Trauma Life Support."

7. ACS-COT, *ATLS Manual*, xxii.

8. Styner, "Guest Editorial: The Birth of Advanced Trauma Life Support."

9. Ibid.

10. ACS-COT, *ATLS Manual*, xxii.

11. Styner, "Guest Editorial: The Birth of Advanced Trauma Life Support."

12. Ryan Corbett Bell, *The Ambulance: A History* (Jefferson, NC: McFarland & Company, 2009), 230, citing a survey conducted by the

American Municipal Association of forty-six cities in which "in a third of the communities, ambulance services were solely managed by private concerns (including for-profit ambulance companies, morticians, and private hospitals)."

13. Ibid., 175.

14. Walt McCall and Tom McPherson, *Classic American Ambulances 1900–1979: Photo Archive* (Hudson, WI: Iconografix, 1999), 91.

15. Bell, *The Ambulance*, 176.

16. McCall and McPherson, *Classic American Ambulances 1900–1979*, 115.

2. THE LESSONS OF WAR

1. Ira M. Rutkow, *Bleeding Blue and Gray* (New York: Random House, 2005), 21. Total casualties, on the Union side alone, numbered 481 dead, 1,011 wounded, and 1,460 missing in action.

2. M. M. Manning, Alan Hawk, Jason H. Calhoun, and Romney C. Andersen, "Treatment of War Wounds: A Historical Review," *Clinical Orthopedics and Related Research* 467, no. 8 (2009): 2168–91, http://www .ncbi.nlm.nih.gov/pmc/articles/PMC2706344.

3. Rutkow, *Bleeding Blue and Gray*, 22–23.

4. W. W. Keen, "Surgical Reminiscences of the Civil War," 1905, reissued in 2015 by Big Byte Books (Amazon Digital Services).

5. Ibid.

6. Shauna Devine, *Learning from the Wounded: The Civil War and the Rise of American Medical Science* (Chapel Hill: University of North Carolina Press, 2014), 6.

7. During the first ten years of the war in Iraq the number of fatalities was about 5,000, and there were an estimated 32,000 wounded. World War II registered 405,399 deaths, World War I 116,516, and Vietnam 58,209. See "Civil War Facts," www.civilwar.org/education/history/faq/, accessed February 6, 2016.

8. Richard A. Gabriel and Karen S. Metz, *A History of Military Medicine*, vol. 2: *From the Renaissance through Modern Times* (New York: Greenwood, 1992), 181.

9. Manning et al., "Treatment of War Wounds," 2180.

10. Gabriel and Metz, *A History of Military Medicine*, 2:182; John T. Greenwood and F. Clifton Berry Jr., *Medics at War: Military Medicine from Colonial Times to the 21st Century* (Annapolis, MD: Association of the U.S. Army, Naval Institute Press, 2005), 30.

11. Frank R. Freeman, *Gangrene and Glory: Medical Care during the*

American Civil War (Cranbury, NJ: Fairleigh Dickinson University Press / Associated University Presses, 1998), 48.

12. E. B. Long, ed., *Personal Memoirs of U. S. Grant* (New York: Da Capo, 1952), 181.

13. Devine, *Learning from the Wounded*, 15.

14. Ibid.

15. Joseph K. Barnes, ed., *The Medical and Surgical History of the War of the Rebellion (1861–1865)* (Washington, DC: U.S. Army Surgeon General's Office, 1870).

16. "The Medical and Surgical History of the War of the Rebellion," Maude Abbot Medical Museum, www.mcgill.ca/medicalmuseum/exhibits /warbones/amm/mshwr, accessed February 1, 2015. See also "Civil War Surgical and Medical Text Books," American Civil War Medicine and Surgical Antiques, www.medicalantiques.com/civilwar/Civil_war_medical _book_collection/Civil_war_medical_books_page_11.htm, accessed February 1, 2015.

17. Rutkow, *Bleeding Blue and Gray*, 106.

18. Ibid., 114.

3. THE WEAKEST LINK

1. Susan P. Baker, "The Stories behind the Statistics," *Injury Epidemiology* 1 (March 2014): 2, www.injepijournal.com/content/1/1/2, accessed February 2, 2016.

2. H. R. Gertner et al., "Evaluation of the Management of Vehicular Fatalities Secondary to Abdominal Injuries," *Journal of Trauma* 12 (1972): 425–31.

3. Robert W. Stock, "Safety Lessons from the Morgue," *New York Times Magazine*, October 26, 2012, www.nytimes.com/2012/10/28/magazine /safety-lessons-from-the-morgue.html.

4. Susan P. Baker, "Fifty Favorites from the Works of Susan P. Baker" (Baltimore: Johns Hopkins Center for Injury Research and Policy, 2012), 2, www.jhsph.edu/research/centers-and-institutes/johns-hopkins-center -for-injury-research-and-policy/50Favs_FINAL-100512.pdf.

5. Baker, "The Stories behind the Statistics," 2.

6. Amy Gangloff, "Safety in Accidents: Hugh DeHaven and the Development of Crash Injury Studies," *Technology and Culture* 54 (January 2013): 40. The author notes that there are conflicting reports regarding whether the other pilot "walked away" or was killed. DeHaven reported in an interview with William Haddon Jr. that the other pilot was killed.

7. David Hemenway, *While We Were Sleeping: Success Stories in Injury and Violence Prevention* (Berkeley: University of California Press, 2009), 20.

8. Ibid., 40.

9. Ibid., 43–45.

10. Hugh DeHaven, "Mechanical Analysis of Survival in Falls from Heights of Fifty to One Hundred and Fifty Feet," *War Medicine* 2 (1942): 586–96.

11. Hemenway, *While We Were Sleeping*, 20.

12. DeHaven, "Mechanical Analysis." According to DeHaven's calculations, the human body tolerated forces up to 200 g, with only trivial injury.

13. Carl Nash, "Hugh DeHaven: Still Relevant for Rollovers," National Crash Analysis Center, presented February 5, 2009, www.sae.org/events /gim/presentations/2009/carlnash.pdf.

14. Griswold and DeHaven applied for the patent in 1951, and it was issued in 1955 as "Combination Shoulder and Lap Safety Belt," Patent No. 2,710,649. It was later further developed by Volvo. USPTO.gov. See also Brian Loebig, "The History of Volvo Seatbelts," April 12, 2013, www .volvoofmidlothian.com/blog/2013/april/13/the-history-of-volvo-seatbelts .htm.

15. Susan P. Baker, "Injury Science Comes of Age," *Journal of the American Medical Association* 262 (1989): 2284–85.

16. Tattoos were not as prevalent as they are today, and the demographic was narrower in the 1970s.

17. William Haddon Jr., "The Changing Approach to the Epidemiology, Prevention, and Amelioration of Trauma: The Transition to Approaches Etiologically Rather Than Descriptively Based," *American Journal of Public Health* 58 (1968): 1431–38.

18. S. P. Baker, L. S. Robertson, and W. U. Spitz, "Tattoos, Alcohol and Violent Death," *Journal of Forensic Sciences* 16 (1971): 190–96.

19. Walter H. Waggoner, "William Haddon Jr., 58, Dies; Authority on Highway Safety, *New York Times*, March 5, 1985, www.nytimes .com/1985/03/05/us/william-haddon-jr-58-dies-authority-on-highway -safety.html.

20. "Medicine: The Fastest Man on Earth," *Time*, September 12, 1955, http://content.time.com/time/subscriber/printout/0,8816,893155,00.html.

21. ACS-COT, *ATLS Student Course Manual*, 284.

22. "Medicine: The Fastest Man on Earth."

23. Ibid.

24. E. Gurdjian, W. Lange, and L. Patrick, eds., *Impact Injury and Crash Protection* (Springfield, IL: Charles C. Thomas, 1970), 312.

25. Ibid., 313.

26. "John Stapp the Human Lab Rat," *Hardcore Heroes*, statement of Samuel Alderson, http://www.history.ca/hardcore-heroes/video /characters/characters-john-stapp/video.html?v=106124867553, accessed April 2, 2015.

27. "Crash Safety Visionary," Stapp Car Crash Conference, www.stapp .org/stapp.shtml, accessed September 2, 2015.

28. "Stapp Car Crash Conference," Stapp Car Crash Conference, www .stapp.org/stapp.shtml, accessed September 2, 2015.

29. Martin A. Croce, David H. Livingston, Frederick A. Luchette, and Robert C. Mackersie, eds., *The American Association for the Surgery of Trauma 75th Anniversary 1938–2013* (Chicago: American Association for the Surgery of Trauma, 2013), 28.

30. Deborah D. Stewart, "More Than Forty Years of Progress for Child Passenger Protection: A Chronicle of Child Passenger Safety Advances in the USA, 1965–2009," *Safe Ride News*, February 2009, http://saferidenews .com/srndnn/LinkClick.aspx?fileticket=NIPfcuqNL1U%3D&tabid=375, accessed February 2, 2016.

31. S. P. Baker and M. W. Lamb, "Hazards of Mountain Flying: Crashes in the Colorado Rockies," *Aviation Space Environmental Medicine* 60 (1989): 531–36.

32. Ibid.

33. Susan P. Baker, "Injury Statistics, High Risk Groups, and Individuals: Falling through the Cracks," an address delivered to Columbia University, Mailman School of Public Health, on May 6, 2010, upon being awarded the Frank A. Calderone Prize in Public Health, https://www.mailman .columbia.edu/sites/default/files/Susan_Baker_Remarks.pdf. In 2010, Baker became the first injury control researcher to be awarded the prize.

34. "Flaura K. Winston," Children's Hospital of Philadelphia, www.chop .edu/doctors/winston-flaura-k#.vkogkWSrTJw, accessed September 2, 2015.

35. Matthew Palumbo, "Spark of Genius: Dr. Janine Jagger Fixes the Problem Not the Blame," *Inventors Eye*, April 2012, www.uspto.gov /custom-page/inventors-eye-dr-janine-jagger-fixes-problem-not-blame.

36. "Runyan Wins APHA Award for Distinguished Career in Injury Control," UNC Gillings School of Global Public Health, November 19,

2014, http://sph.unc.edu/sph-news/runyan-wins-apha-award-for-distinguished-career-in-injury-control/, accessed February 2, 2016.

4. LEARNING TO FLY

1. "His Aviation Firsts," Igor Sikorsky Historical Archives, updated November 6, 2012, www.sikorskyarchives.com/His_Aviation_Firsts%20R1 .php, accessed February 6, 2016.

2. "S-47-R4 Helicopter," Igor Sikorsky Historical Archives, updated November 6, 2012, www.sikorskyarchives.com/S-47.php., accessed February 6, 2016.

3. Robert F. Dorr, *Chopper: Firsthand Accounts of Helicopter Warfare, World War II to Iraq* (New York: Berkley, 2005), 17.

4. Ibid., 10. Dorr states that on the first test flight undertaken overseas in India a YR-4B crashed, killing the pilot and crew.

5. Ibid., 2.

6. Ibid., 4.

7. Ibid., 8.

8. "Training Fact Sheet: Density Altitude," International Helicopter Safety Team, www.ihst.org/Portals/54/insights/Density_Altitude.pdf, accessed February 6, 2016. According to this fact sheet, heat and humidity affect density altitude, simulating high altitude conditions and adversely affecting helicopter performance.

9. Friends of the Helicopter Museum, "Celebrating the 65th Anniversary, on 25th April 2009 of the First Helicopter Rescue," www.hmfriends .org.uk/combatrescue65th.htm, accessed February 6, 2016. This article states that after the war, the pilot of the first helicopter rescue in the history of the armed forces went on to distinguish himself further as a composer, music critic for the *New York Times* and *Time* magazine, author (*A Popular History of Music from Gregorian Chant to Jazz*), and record producer.

10. The H-13 had a long fuselage and an oversized bubble canopy, hence the nickname "grasshopper."

11. Darryl Whitcomb, *Call Sign—Dustoff: A History of U.S. Army Aeromedical Evacuation from Conception to Hurricane Katrina* (Frederick, MD: Office of the Surgeon General, Borden Institute, 2011), 17.

12. Ibid., 22.

13. Spurgeon H. Neel Jr., "Medical Considerations in Helicopter Evacuation," *U.S. Armed Forces Medical Journal* 5, no. 2 (February 1954): 221. Neel was awarded the Purple Heart for his World War II wounds.

14. Ibid., 221.

15. Whitcomb, *Call Sign—Dustoff*, 26.

16. Ibid. The nickname "Huey" derives from the initial HU-1 designation, which was later changed to UH-1.

17. Ibid., 68.

18. John L. Cook, *Rescue under Fire: The Story of Dust Off in Vietnam* (Atglen, PA: Schiffer Military/Aviation History, 1998), 44.

19. The American Red Cross, "Summary of the Geneva Conventions of 1949 and Their Additional Protocols," April 2011, www.redcross .org/images/MEDIA_CustomProductCatalog/m3640104_IHL _SummaryGenevaConv.pdf.

20. Dorr, *Chopper*, 248.

21. Cook, *Rescue under Fire*, 59.

22. Ibid., 65–69.

23. Ibid., 82.

24. Triple-canopy jungles are those with three layers of overhead vegetation of increasing heights, measuring up to fifty feet. "Definition of Common Terms," www.134thahc.com/Definitions.htm, accessed February 6, 2016.

25. Cook, *Rescue under Fire*, 94–96. For a diagram and photos of the Jungle Penetrator, see *Search and Rescue: Jungle Penetrator*, www.cc.gatech .edu/~tpilsch/AirOps/sar-penetrator.html., accessed February 6, 2016.

26. Peter Dorland and James Nanney, *Dust Off: Army Aeromedical Evacuation in Vietnam* (Washington, DC: Center of Military History, U.S. Army, 1982), 72.

27. Dorr, *Chopper*, 250–53.

28. Bell, *The Ambulance*, 170.

29. Ibid., 171.

30. "History of Air Medical and Air Ambulance Services in the United States," Air Ambulance Guides, August 21, 2012, www.airambulanceguides .com/history-of-air-medical-and-air-ambulance-services-in-the-united -states/.

31. Ibid.

32. Bell, *The Ambulance*, 172.

5. RESCUE WARRIORS

1. Jenifer Goodwin, "How Pittsburgh's 'Freedom House' Shaped Modern EMS Systems," EMS1.com, January 31, 2014, www.ems1.com /best-practices/articles/1977832-How-Pittsburghs-Freedom-House -shaped-modern-EMS-systems/.

2. Bell, *The Ambulance*, 257.

3. "Lawrence Just Slips Away," *Pittsburgh Post-Gazette*, November 22, 1966, https://news.google.com/newspapers?id=aosqAAAAIBAJ&sjid=pk8EAAAAIBAJ&pg=7427%2C2875765.

4. Manish N. Shah, "The Formation of the Emergency Medical Services System," *American Journal of Public Health* 96 (2006): 2, www.ncbi.nlm.nih.gov/pmc/articles/PMC1470509.

5. Goodwin, "How Pittsburgh's 'Freedom House' Shaped Modern EMS Systems."

6. Ibid.

7. Bell, *The Ambulance*, 258.

8. Lisa Vox, "Timeline of the Civil Rights Movement," About.com, http://afroamhistory.about.com/od/timelines/a/timelinelate60s.htm, accessed March 1, 2015.

9. Robyn Meredith, "5 Days in 1967 Still Shake Detroit," *New York Times*, July 23, 1997, www.nytimes.com/1997/07/23/us/5-days-in-1967-still-shake-detroit.html?pagewanted=1.

10. Emily Ruby, "1968: The Year That Rocked Pittsburgh," *Western Pennsylvania History* (Spring 2013), http://journals.psu.edu/wph/article/viewFile/59171/58896.

11. Anita Srikameswaran, "Dr. Peter Safar: A Life Devoted to Cheating Death," *Pittsburgh Post-Gazette*, March 31, 2002, http://old.post-gazette.com/lifestyle/20020331safar0331fnp2.asp.

12. Ibid.

13. "Obituary: Peter J. Safar," *Resuscitation* 59 (2003): 4.

14. Bell, *The Ambulance*, 252.

15. Ibid.

16. J. D. Farrington, "Death in a Ditch," *American College of Surgeons Bulletin* 52 (June 1967): 121.

17. Ibid., 123.

18. Bell, *The Ambulance*, 263.

19. Ibid., 268.

20. This was a relatively simple fix: an inverter was added to convert the defibrillator's power source from alternating current (from an outlet) to direct current supplied by batteries.

21. Mark Peck, "Professor Frank Pantridge," EMSMuseum.org, www.emsmuseum.org/virtual-museum/by_era/articles/399784-Professor-Frank-Pantridge, accessed April 1, 2015.

22. J. F. Pantridge and J. S. Geddes, "Mobile Intensive-Care Unit in the Management of Myocardial Infarction," *The Lancet*, August 5, 1967, 271.

23. Barry Shurlock, "Pioneers in Cardiology: Frank Pantridge, CBE, MC, MD, FRCP, FACC," *Circulation* 25 (2007): f145, http://circ.ahajournals.org /content/116/25/F145.full.pdf, accessed February 6, 2016.

24. "Pioneers of Paramedicine Inaugural Honorees," Los Angeles County Fire Museum, www.pioneersofparamedicine.com/Pioneers.html, accessed April 1, 2015.

25. Bell, *The Ambulance*, 293.

26. Susan Gilmore, "Rusty Motor Home Part of Medic One's History," *Seattle Times*, November 29, 2011, www.seattletimes.com/seattle-news /rusty-motor-home-part-of-medic-ones-history/.

27. G. S. Fortner, M. R. Oreskovich, M. K. Copass, and C. J. Carrico, "The Effects of Prehospital Trauma Care on Survival from a 50-Meter Fall," *Journal of Trauma* 23, no. 11 (1983): 976–81.

28. Bell, *The Ambulance*, 295.

29. "1976: Nancy Caroline MD," Virtual EMS Museum, www .emsmuseum.org/virtual-museum/publications/articles/398276-1976 -Nancy-Caroline-MD, accessed April 15, 2015. Known as the "Orange Book," *Emergency Care in the Streets* was the first manual of prehospital care and is now in its seventh edition (the fortieth anniversary edition was published in 2012).

30. Lisa Dionne, "The Untold Story of EMS Response to the World Trade Center Attack on Sept. 11," in *Courage under Fire*, suppl. to *Journal of Emergency Medical Services* (September 2002), www.jems.com/articles /supplements/special-topics/courage-under-fire.html.

31. Ibid. The eight EMS personnel who died on September 11, 2001, were Keith Fairben (EMT-P, New York Presbyterian Hospital EMS), Carlos Lillo (FDNY paramedic), Yamel Merino (EMT, MetroCare Ambulance), Richard Pearlman (volunteer, Forest Hills Volunteer Ambulance Corp.), Ricardo Quinn (FDNY paramedic), Mario Santoro (EMT-P, New York Presbyterian Hospital EMS), Mark Schwartz (EMT, Hunter Ambulance), and David Marc Sullins (EMT, Cabrini Hospital EMS).

32. Bell, *The Ambulance*, 271.

33. Nicole Norfleet, "St. Paul Fire EMTs Provide CPR Training," *Minneapolis Star Tribune*, April 23, 2015, www.startribune.com/st-paul -fire-emts-provide-CPR-training/301150701, accessed February 6, 2016.

34. Bell, *The Ambulance*, 275.

35. Goodwin, "How Pittsburgh's 'Freedom House' Shaped Modern EMS Systems."

36. Ibid.

6. HURT

1. Jon Franklin and Alan Doelp, *Shock-Trauma* (New York: St. Martin's, 1980), 6.

2. As noted in ibid., R Adams Cowley's birth certificate reads R (no period) Adams Cowley.

3. Frederick Heaton Millham, "A Brief History of Shock," *Surgery* 148 (2010): 1034.

4. There is more than one type of shock. I am focusing on hypovolemic shock, i.e., shock due to low blood volume or dehydration, the most common type that arises in trauma patients. Shock may also occur secondary to severe infection, cardiac malfunction, and spinal cord injury or disease, in which case the symptoms may vary from the classic triad.

5. Thomas M. Scalea, "R Adams Cowley," *Trauma* 17 (2015): 77.

6. Franklin and Doelp, *Shock-Trauma*, 19–21.

7. Ibid., 7.

8. Ibid., 21.

9. Ibid., 17.

10. Ibid., 31.

11. "Mobile Surgical Units Prevent Delays in Treating Wounded Combat Patients in Iraq," *Science Daily*, January 28, 2005, www.sciencedaily.com /releases/2005/01/050126111737.htm.

12. Franklin and Doelp, *Shock-Trauma*, 71.

13. Ibid., 73.

14. Ibid., 75.

15. Thomas M. Scalea, "R Adams Cowley," *Trauma* 17 (2015): 78.

16. Richard J. Mullins, "A Historical Perspective of Trauma System Development in the United States," *Journal of Trauma* 3 (1991): S8–S14, http:// ipsapp003.lwwonline.com/content/getfile/2281/75/4/fulltext.htm.

17. Ibid.

18. David R. Boyd, "How Illinois' Trauma and EMS System of Care Helped Shape the Industry," *Journal of Emergency Medical Services* 40, no. 3 (March 30, 2015), www.jems.com/articles/print/volume-40/issue-3 /features/road-professionalism.html.

19. A. Brent Eastman, "Wherever the Dart Lands: Toward the Ideal Trauma System," *Journal of the American College of Surgeons* 5, Appendix

G (2010): 156, http://www.emsa.ca.gov/Media/Default/Word /2014TraumaPlanForComment/G_APPENDIX_Scudder_Oration.pdf., accessed February 5, 2016.

20. Martin A. Croce, David H. Livingston, Frederick A. Luchette, and Robert C. Mackersie, eds., *The American Association for the Surgery of Trauma 75th Anniversary 1938–2013* (The American Association for the Surgery of Trauma, 2013), 327 (an interview with F. William Blaisdell, MD, President, 1990–91).

21. Moishe Liberman, David S. Mulder, and John S. Sampalis, "The History of Trauma Care Systems from Homer to Telemedicine," *McGill Journal of Medicine* (2004), accessed March 3, 2015.

22. "Access to Trauma Centers in the United States," U.S. Department of Health and Human Services Centers for Disease Control and Prevention, September 2009, www.cdc.gov/TraumaCare.

23. Trauma centers are classified as Levels I–III. Level I centers provide the highest level of care.

24. Jason Silverstein, "The Decline of Emergency Care," *Atlantic*, April 2013, www.theatlantic.com/health/archive/2013/04/the-decline-of -emergency-care/275306.

25. Robert J. Schoderbek, Todd C. Battaglia, Erik R. Dorf, and David M. Kahler, "Traumatic Hemipelvectomy: Case Report and Literature Review," *The Archives of Orthopedic Trauma Surgery* 125 (2005): 360.

26. Ibid., 361.

27. Hugh Foy, email to the author, April 24, 2015.

28. "Alloderm Tissue Matrix Defined," LifeCell.com, www.lifecell.com /health-care-professionals/lifecell-products/allodermr-regenerative-tissue -matrix/allodermr-tissue-matrix-defined/ (accessed August 19, 2015).

29. Michelle Reichert, "Back in the Saddle," *Belgrade News*, November 20, 2010, www.belgrade-news.com/features/article_9688ee98-f41f-11df -afb4-001cc4c002e0.html, accessed March 10, 2015.

30. Michael Rosenwald, "Yesterday They Would Have Died," *Popular Science*, October 2003, 61.

31. Suzanne Wooton, "Man Who Saved So Many from Death Is Buried: Dr. R Adams Cowley Bid Emotional Farewell," *Baltimore Sun*, November 5, 1991, http://articles.baltimoresun.com/1991-11-05/news/1991309018 _1_r-adams-cowley-shock-trauma-trauma-center. See also Trauma Net: Trauma Centers, www.maryland-traumanet.com/about-network /trauma-centers/.

7. THE COLOR OF BLOOD

1. S.v. "exsanguination," *Oxford English Dictionary*, http://www
.oxforddictionaries.com/us/definition/american_english/exsanguination,
accessed February 4, 2016.

2. Alison Kabaroff, "Stop the Bleeding," *Journal of Emergency Medical
Services*, November 7, 2013, www.jems.com/print/29694.

3. Shawn C. Nessen, Dave E. Lounsbury, and Stephen P. Hetz, eds., *War
Surgery in Afghanistan and Iraq: A Series of Cases, 2003–2007* (Washington,
DC: Office of the Surgeon General, Borden Institute, Walter Reed Army
Medical Center, 2008), 39.

4. H. C. Tien et al., "Preventable Deaths from Hemorrhage at a Level I
Canadian Trauma Center," *Journal of Trauma* 62, no. 1 (January 2007):
142–46.

5. U. Katzenell et al., "Analysis of the Causes of Death of Casualties in
Field Military Setting," *Military Medicine* 177, no. 9 (2012): 1065–68.

6. Nessen, Lounsbury, and Hetz, *War Surgery*, 289.

7. The military follows MARCH guidelines for combat resuscitation:
Massive hemorrhage, Airway, Respirations, Circulation and Hypothermia. Kabaroff, "Stop the Bleeding."

8. Nessen, Lounsbury, and Hetz, *War Surgery*, 289, stating that
applying a tourniquet before a patient goes into shock improves survival
by 90 percent.

9. Ibid., 288.

10. "What Is QuikClot?," www.quikclot.com/About-QuikClot, accessed
February 3, 2016.

11. Todd Leopold, "Tool Can Plug Gunshot Wounds in Seconds," CNN
.com, June 2, 2014, www.cnn.com/2014/06/02/tech/innovation/xstat
-wound-treatment.

12. Nessen, Lounsbury, and Hetz, *War Surgery*, 42–43.

13. "Blood Facts and Statistics," American Red Cross, April 3, 2015, www
.redcrossblood.org/print/learn-about-blood/blood-facts-and-statistics.

14. "M. D. Anderson Blood Bank," University of Texas M. D. Anderson
Cancer Center, www.mdanderson.org/how-you-can-help/donate-blood
/index.html, accessed February 3, 2016.

15. Spencie Love, *One Blood: The Death and Resurrection of Charles R.
Drew* (Chapel Hill: University of North Carolina Press, 1996), 145.

16. Ibid.

17. Ibid., 146.

18. Ibid., 148.

19. "The Charles R. Drew Papers: Biographical Information," Profiles in Science, The National Library of Medicine, Bethesda, MD, http://profiles .nlm.nih.gov/ps/retrieve/Narrative/Bg/p-nid/336, accessed April 10, 2015.

20. Love, *One Blood*, 116–19.

21. "The Charles R. Drew Papers: Becoming 'the Father of the Blood Bank,'" Profiles in Science, The National Library of Medicine, Bethesda, MD, http://profiles.nlm.nih.gov/ps/retrieve/Narrative/Bg/p-nid/336, accessed April 10, 2015.

22. Drew's thesis, "Banked Blood: A Study in Blood Preservation," can be found at http://profiles.nlm.nih.gov/ps/access/BGBBJT.pdf (accessed January 21, 2016).

23. Love, *One Blood*, 152.

24. Ibid., 155.

25. Ibid., 158.

26. Ibid., 170.

27. Ibid., 172.

28. Jason H. Gart, "Interview with Dr. LaSalle D. Leffall, Jr., November 19, 2010," Digital Manuscripts Program of the National Library of Medicine Oral History Project, http://profiles.nlm.nih.gov/ps/access/bgbbjv.pdf.

29. Nina Notman, "Artificial Blood: Synthetic Alternatives to Donor Blood Have Been Stuck in Development for Decades," *Chemistry World* (October 2010): 40, www.chemistryworld.org.

30. Eric Adler, "Kansas Jehovah's Witness Saved by Blood Substitute," *Topeka Capital-Journal*, May 6, 2013, http://cjonline.come/news/2013-05 -06/kansas-jehovahs-witness-saved-blood-substitute.

31. Notman, "Artificial Blood," 42.

32. Ibid.

8. A TOWER OF TERROR

1. Gary M. Lavergne, *A Sniper in the Tower* (Denton: University of North Texas Press, 1997), 132.

2. Ibid., 143.

3. One of the wounded, David Gumby, had to be on dialysis for kidney failure after the shootings. He died in 2001, and his death was ruled a homicide. Baby boy Wilson was not counted as one of the fatalities, although at eight months of gestation he was viable and would be counted today. The total death count including both would be eighteen. See "Victim of UT Shooting Dies after 30 Years," *Texas Landmarks and Legacies*, November 7, 2011, http://howdyyall.com/Texas/TodaysNews/index.cfm?getItem=988.

4. Pamela Coloff, "96 Minutes," *Texas Monthly*, August 2006, www
.texasmonthly.com/articles/96-minutes/.

5. The equation for determining force (*F*) involves mass (*m*) and velocity
(*v*): $F = \frac{1}{2}\,m \times v^2$.

6. Lavergne, *A Sniper in the Tower*, 144.

7. Ibid., 160.

8. Ibid., 169.

9. A bronze plaque memorializing the victims was placed in the
University of Texas Tower garden on January 10, 2007, forty-one years
later. "Memorial Plaque in Tower Garden Commemorates Victims of Aug.
1, 1966 Shooting Tragedy," *UT News*, January 10, 2007, http://news.utexas
.edu/2007/01/10/tower_garden.

10. Diane Cecilia Weber, "Warrior Cops: The Ominous Growth of
Paramilitarism in American Police Departments," Cato Institute Briefing
Papers, August 26, 1999, http://object.cato.org/sites/cato.org/files/pubs
/pdf/bp50.pdf.

11. Radley Balko, "Rise of the Warrior Cop," *Wall Street Journal*, August
7, 2013, www.wsj.com/articles/SB10001424127887323848048045786080407
80519904.

12. Austin Police Department, "Special Weapons and Tactics (SWAT)
Team," September 3, 2015, https://www.austintexas.gov/department/
special-weapons-and-tactics-swat-team.

13. Joseph A. Califano Jr., "Gun Control Lessons from Lyndon Johnson,"
Washington Post, December 16, 2012, https://www.washingtonpost.com
/opinions/gun-control-lessons-from-lyndon-johnson/2012/12/16
/38f3941e-47b4-11e2-ad54-580638ede391_story.html?hpid=z2.

14. Ibid.

15. Samantha Michaels, "The United States Has Had More Mass
Shootings Than Any Other Country," *Mother Jones*, August 23, 2015, www
.motherjones.com/print/282386.

16. "U.S. Gun Violence: History of Deadly Shootings," *Sky News*, October
2, 2015, http://news.sky.com/story/1562458/us-gun-violence-history-of
-deadly-shootings.

17. There is no official definition of a mass shooting. Some define
mass shootings as four or more shot and estimate the number during the
Obama administration to number in the hundreds: Philip Bump, "The San
Bernardino Shooting Continues a Disturbing Trend: No Week since 2013
without a Mass Shooting," *Washington Post*, December 2, 2015, www
.washingtonpost.com/news/the-fix/wp/2015/10/01/theres-been-no

-calendar-week-without-a-mass-shooting-during-president-obamas
-second-term/. I am using the FBI definition of four or more killings in
a public setting: Mark Follman, "How Many Mass Shootings Are There,
Really?," *New York Times*, December 3, 2015, http://www.nytimes.com
/2015/12/04/opinion/how-many-mass-shootings-are-there-really.html.

18. Gardiner Harris and Michael D. Shear, "Obama Condemns 'Routine'
of Mass Shootings, Says U.S. Has Become Numb," *New York Times*, October
1, 2015.

19. Dan Turkel, "More Americans Have Died in the Last Year from Gun
Violence Than in the Last 40 Years from Terror Attacks," *Business Insider*,
October 1, 2015, www.businessinsider.com/more-americans-have-die
-from-gun-violence-than-terror-attacks-2015-10.

20. Liat Clark, "U.S. Mass Shootings Blamed on High Gun Ownership
and 'American Dream,'" *Wired*, August 24, 2015, http://www.wired.co
.uk/news/archive/2015-08/24/gun-ownership-mass-shootings-us-study,
accessed February 4, 2016.

21. Erik Eckholm, "Rampage Killings Linger in Memory, but Toll of Gun
Violence Is Constant," *New York Times*, October 8, 2015, www.nytimes
.com/2015/10/09/us/rampage-killings-get-attention-but-gun-violence-is
-constant.html?_r=0.

22. Audie Cornish interview with Jack Levin, "Many Mass Killers Have
Had Chronic Depression," *All Things Considered*, NPR, December 14, 2012,
www.npr.org/2012/12/14/167287373/many-mass-killers-have-had-chronic
-depression.

23. Christopher Ingraham, "This Is What One Year of Gun Deaths in
America Looks Like," *Washington Post*, October 2, 2015, www
.washingtonpost.com/news/wonkblog/wp/2015/10/14/people-are
-getting-shot-by-toddlers-on-a-weekly-basis-this-year/.

24. Daniel Webster, "America's Path to Fewer Gun Deaths," presentation delivered at TEDMED, September 10, 2014, www.jhsph.edu/research
/centers-and-institutes/johns-hopkins-center-for-gun-policy-and
-research/daniel-webster-tedmed-talk.html.

25. Roger Parloff, "Smart Guns? They're Ready. Are We?" *Fortune*,
April 22, 2015, http://fortune.com/2015/04/22/smart-guns-theyre-ready
-are-we/.

26. Christopher Ingraham, "People Are Getting Shot by Toddlers on
a Weekly Basis This Year," *Washington Post*, October 14, 2015, www
.washingtonpost.com/news/wonkblog/wp/2015/10/14/people-are
-getting-shot-by-toddlers-on-a-weekly-basis-this-year/.

27. Webster, "America's Path to Fewer Gun Deaths."

28. Carolyn Tyler, "San Francisco's Last Gun Shop to Close as Supervisors Pass Gun Control Measure," ABC7News.Com, October 27, 2015, http://abc7news.com/politics/sfs-last-gun-shop-to-close-as-supervisors-pass-gun-control-measure/1053935/.

29. Sheryl Gay Stolberg, "Oregon Killings Amplify Crusade of Virginia Tech Victim's Father," New York Times, October 10, 2015 (video of Joseph Samaha speaking), www.nytimes.com/2015/10/11/us/oregon-killings-amplify-crusade-of-virginia-tech-victims-father.html.

30. Christine Hauser, "Families of Virginia Tech Massacre Victims Start Program to Improve Campus Safety," New York Times, August 13, 2015, www.nytimes.com/2015/08/14/us/virginia-tech-massacre-victims-national-campus-safety-initiative.html.

31. Andrew Roush, "Whitman Shooting Lingers over Campus Carry Debate," Alcalde: The Official Publication of the Texas Exes, February 22, 2015, http://alcalde.texasexes.org/2015/02/whitman-shooting-lingers-over-campus-carry-debate/.

32. Lauren R. McGaughy, "Whitman Victim Testifies against Open-Carry Gun Bill," Houston Chronicle, February 12, 2015, www.chron.com/about/article/Whitman-victim-testifies-against-open-carry-6077967.php. Claire Wilson, aka Claire James, was the first victim to be shot from the Tower. Five others were shot inside the Tower on the twenty-seventh floor before she was shot.

33. McGaughy, "Whitman Victim Testifies."

34. Manny Fernandez and Dave Montgomery, "Texas Lawmakers Pass a Bill Allowing Guns at Colleges," New York Times, June 2, 2015, www.nytimes.com/2015/06/03/us/texas-lawmakers-approve-bill-allowing-guns-on-campus.html?_r=0. This article notes that Texas joins seven other states (Colorado, Kansas, Utah, Idaho, Oregon, Mississippi, and Wisconsin) in allowing guns on campuses.

9. OFF-ROAD MD

1. The Other Shore: The Diana Nyad Story, dir. Timothy Wheeler, Doc Life Films, 2013.

2. Albert H. Meinke, Jr., MD, Mountain Troops and Medics: Wartime Stories of a Frontline Surgeon in the U.S. Ski Troops (Kewadin, MI: Rucksack Publishing, 1993), 100.

3. Ibid., 99.

4. David C. Cone, Jane H. Brice, Theodore R. Delbridge, and J. Brent

Myers, eds., *Emergency Medical Services: Clinical Practice and Systems Oversight*, 2nd ed. (West Sussex, England: John Wiley & Sons, 2015), 379.

5. "Outdoor Emergency Care," Timber Ridge Ski Patrol, www.trskipatrol.org/outdoor-emergency-care, accessed February 5, 2016.

6. Marie Griffin, "Tough Mudder Is Finding Its Stride, And It Has No Plans to Slow Down," *SmartCEO.com*, http://smartceo.com/tough-mudder-finding-stride-no-plans-slow/, accessed February 5, 2016.

7. Claudia Dreifus, "A Conversation with Kenneth Kamler; Bringing Them Back, Healthy, from the Ends of the Earth," *New York Times*, June 22, 2004, www.nytimes.com/2004/06/22/health/conversation-with-kenneth-kamler-bringing-them-back-healthy-ends-earth.html?pagewanted=all.

8. Ibid.

9. Ibid.

10. Kenneth Kamler, "My Mount Everest Story," *Huffington Post*, February 3, 2014, www.huffingtonpost.com/kenneth-kamler/my-mount-everest-story_b_4719831.html.

11. Dreifus, "A Conversation with Kenneth Kamler."

12. Raymond B. Huey and Xavier Eguskitza, "Limits to Human Performance: Elevated Risks on High Mountains," *Journal of Experimental Biology* 204 (2001), http://jeb.biolgists.org/content/204/18/3115.long.

13. Molly Loomis, "Inside the ER at Mt. Everest," *Smithsonian*, May 31, 2011, www.smithsonianmag.com/ist/?next=/people-places/inside-the-er-at-mt-everest-180237745/.

14. Ed Douglas, "My Life after Death," *The Guardian*, October 21, 2000, www.theguardian.com/theobserver/2000/oct/22/focus.news.

15. Jesse Greenspan, "7 Things You Should Know about Mount Everest," *History.com*, May 29, 2013, www.history.com/news/7-things-you-should-know-about-mount-everest.

16. Everest South Side (Nepal) Camps, *Everest News*, www.everestnews.com/everestnews/camps.htm, accessed February 5, 2016. Climbers spend time at five Mount Everest camps. Base camp at 17,500 feet is where the support staff, including medical personnel, are stationed. It is also where climbers typically acclimate for several weeks. Camp I is at 19,500 feet. Camp II is at 21,000 feet. Camp III is at 23,700 feet. To get to Camp III, climbers must climb a sheer wall of ice, the Lhotse Face. Camp IV, or High Camp, located in the Death Zone, is at 26,300 feet. The summit, the highest peak on earth, is at 29,028 feet.

17. Beck Weathers, *Left for Dead* (New York: Villard Books, 2000), 32.

18. Ibid., 37–50.

19. Benjamin C. Wedro and William C. Shiel Jr., "Frostbite and Hypothermia Symptoms and Stages," emedicinehealth.com, www.emedicinehealth.com/script/main/art.asp?articlekey=124962, accessed February 5, 2016.

20. Eric Benson, "After Everest: The Complete Story of Beck Weathers," *Men's Journal*, September 2015, www.mensjournal.com/essential/print-view/after-everest-the-complete-story-of-beck-weathers-20150909.

21. Weathers, *Left for Dead*, 53–54.

22. Kalmer, "My Mount Everest Story."

23. Ibid.

24. *Field Guide to Wilderness Medicine*, 3rd ed. (Philadelphia: Moby Elsevier, 2008), 34–36.

25. Ibid.

26. Hawaiian Box Jelly page, Pacific Cnidaria Research Lab, http://www5.pbrc.hawaii.edu/pcrl/research.html, accessed February 5, 2016. See also Cedric M. Yshimotot and Angel Anne Yanagihara, "Cnidarian (Coelenterate) Envenomations in Hawai'i Improve Following Heat Application," *Transactions of the Royal Society of Tropical Medicine and Hygiene* 96 (2002): 300.

27. Eric A. Weiss, "Backcountry 911: 1,001 Uses for Duct Tape and Safety Pins," presented at the 2009 American College of Emergency Physicians Scientific Assembly, October 16, 2011, San Francisco, CA, http://acep.omnibooksonline.com/Boston2009/data/papers/WE-168.pdf.

28. Lloyd Vries, "Climber Describes Amputation Ordeal," CBS News, May 2, 2003, www.cbsnews.com/news/climber-describes-amputation-ordeal/.

29. Christopher Reynolds, "Arizona: At the Grand Canyon, 683 Scary Stories, All True," *Los Angeles Times*, March 19, 2012, http://articles.latimes.com/2012/mar/19/news/la-trb-death-grand-canyon-20120315.

30. John Branch, "Lost Brother in Yosemite," *New York Times*, June 14, 2015, 1.

31. Michael P. Ghiglieri and Thomas M. Myers, *Over the Edge: Death in the Grand Canyon*, 14th rev. (Flagstaff, AZ: Puma Press, 2001), 20.

32. Cyndy Cole, "Canyon Deaths: 685 and Counting," *Arizona Daily Sun*, May 6, 2012, http://azdailysun.com/news/local/canyon-deaths-and-counting/article_ba588a05-e816-55be-87f6-80f15b76f744.html.

33. Ibid.

34. Cyndy Cole, "Fatal Fall Ends Canyon Dream," *Arizona Daily Sun*, May 6, 2012, http://azdailysun.com/news/local/fatal-fall-ends-canyon-dream/article_c4b475df-ea5d-546d-9fef-1095d3d31c8d.html.

35. Brandon Bowers, "Two Hikers Killed in Separate Incidents at Yosemite National Park," *Merced Sun-Star*, May 16, 2011, www.mercedsunstar.com /news/local/community/mariposa-and-yosemite/article3259488.html.

36. Lennox H. Huang, "Dehydration Clinical Presentation," *Medscape*, December 31, 2015, http://emedicine.medscape.com/article/906999 -clinical#b4.

37. "Sports Medicine Team Witnesses Diana Nyad's Determination," *University of Miami Miller School of Medicine News*, October 6, 2011, http:// med.miami.edu/news/sports-medicine-team-witnesses-diana-nyads -determination.

38. *The Other Shore: The Diana Nyad Story*, dir. Timothy Wheeler, Doc Life Films, 2013.

39. Fitz Cahall, "Diana Nyad—Adventurers of the Year 2014," *National Geographic*, http://adventure.nationalgeographic.com/adventure /adventurers-of-the-year/2014/diana-nyad/, accessed August 15, 2015. Nyad's first attempt was in 1978. The next four attempts took place from 2011 to 2013. Clifton Page, email to author, October 7, 2014.

40. "In the News: UHMed Jellyfish Expert Dr. Angel Yanagihara Assists Diana Nyad in Historic Swim," *UH Med Now Newsletter*, September 4, 2013, http://jabsom.hawaii.edu/in-the-news-uhmed-jellyfish-expert-dr-angel -yanagihara-assists-diana-nyad-in-historic-swim/. See also Diana Nyad, "Box Jellyfish—Deadly Venom," *Huffpost Green*, last updated September 3, 2013, www.huffingtonpost.com/diana-nyad/box-jellyfish-deadly-veno_b _3546799.html.

41. Samantha Bonar, "Diana Nyad's Jellyfish-Proof Secret Weapon? A Prosthetics Expert in Altadena," *LA Weekly*, September 6, 2013, www .laweekly.com/arts/diana-nyads-jellyfish-proof-secret-weapon-a -prosthetics-expert-in-altadena-4184622.

42. "Miller School Team Supports Diana Nyad's Marathon Swim," *University of Miami Miller School of Medicine News*, September 10, 2013, http://med.miami.edu/news/miller-school-team-supports-diana-nyads -marathon-swim.

10. THE SAVE

1. C. J. Williams, "Harold Gillies: Aesthetic Reconstructor," *The New Zealand Edge: Heroes*, June 26, 2002, http://www.nzedge.com/legends /harold-gillies/.

2. Andrew Bamji, "Sir Harold Gillies: Surgical Pioneer," *Trauma* 8, no. 3 (July 2006): 143.

3. Ibid., 144.

4. Ibid.

5. David J. Brain, "Facial Surgery during World War I," *Facial Plastic Surgery* 9 (April 1993): 159.

6. In 1798, French surgeon Pierre Desault dubbed the techniques used to repair facial deformities "plastic surgery," from the Greek *plasticos* (fit for molding). Early plastic techniques can be traced back to 600 B.C., when a Hindu surgeon fashioned a nose from a piece of cheek. In the sixteenth century, Italian surgeon Gaspare Tagliacozzi used flaps of upper arm skin to reconstruct noses slashed off in sword fights.

7. Brain, "Facial Surgery," 159.

8. Olga Khazan, "Masks: The Face Transplant of World War I," *Atlantic*, August 4, 2014, www.theatlantic.com/health/archive/2014/08/the-first -face-transplants-were-masks/375527/.

9. Ibid.

10. Ibid.

11. Ibid., 146.

12. Harold D. Gillies, *Plastic Surgery of the Face: Based on Selected Cases of War Injuries of the Face Including Burns* (London: Oxford University Press, 1920), 168.

13. Ibid., 170–71.

14. George W. Pierce and Gerald B. O'Conner, "The Tubed Pedicle Flap in Reconstruction Surgery," *California and Western Medicine* 62, no. 1 (August 1931): 94.

15. A photograph of a tube pedicle flap and more about Gillies can be found at this BBC website: "Faces of Battle," *BBC News*, http://news.bbc.co .uk/2/shared/spl/hi/picture_gallery/07/magazine_faces_of_battle/html /6.stm, accessed February 5, 2016.

16. The first tube pedicle flap was allegedly constructed by Professor V. P. Gilatov of the Novororssiisk Eye Clinic in Odessa, Ukraine, on September 9, 1916, but Gillies was unaware of it and created his version independently. Brain, "Facial Surgery," 162.

17. Liza Gross, "New Hope for Soldiers Disfigured in War," *Discover*, September 2014, http://discovermagazine.com/2014/sept/11-face-of-hope.

18. Claudia Dreifus, "Healing Soldiers' Most Exposed Wounds," *New York Times*, December 2, 2013, www.nytimes.com/2013/12/03/science /healing-soldiers-most-exposed-wounds.html.

19. Gross, "New Hope for Soldiers Disfigured in War."

20. Ibid.

21. Dreifus, "Healing Soldiers' Most Exposed Wounds."

22. Gross, "New Hope for Soldiers Disfigured in War."

23. Dreifus, "Healing Soldiers' Most Exposed Wounds."

24. Gross, "New Hope for Soldiers Disfigured in War."

11. OUR PLASTIC BRAINS

1. Lee Woodruff and Bob Woodruff, *In an Instant: A Family's Journey of Love and Healing* (New York: Random House, 2007), 238. Woodruff discusses *ABC World News Tonight* anchor Peter Jennings, who had spent eighteen years as a foreign correspondent before becoming a network anchor.

2. Ibid., 22.

3. Malcolm W. Nance, *The Terrorists of Iraq: Inside the Strategy and Tactics of the Iraq Insurgency 2003–2014*, 2nd ed. (Boca Raton, FL: CRC Press, Taylor & Francis Group, 2015), 149.

4. Woodruff and Woodruff, *In an Instant*, 22–23.

5. "BIAA Adopts New Definition," Brain Injury Association of America, February 6, 2011, www.biausa.org/announcements/biaa-adopts-new-tbi -definition.

6. "Where Soldiers Come From: Traumatic Brain Injury," *POV*, PBS.org, November 11, 2011, www.pbs.org/pov/wheresoldierscomefrom/traumatic -brain-injury.php. Estimates (through November 2011) of the number of soldiers with TBI from the Iraq and Afghanistan wars vary widely depending on source, from fifty thousand (Department of Defense) to four hundred thousand (the Rand Corporation). See also Erin Bagalman, "Traumatic Brain Injury among Veterans," *Congressional Research Service*, January 4, 2013, www.ncbi.nlm.nih.gov/pubmed/22776913. Bagalman states that it may be impossible to know the true number, as soldiers from early deployments were probably underdiagnosed and mild TBIs may be misdiagnosed as PTSD.

7. Erin Bagalman, "Traumatic Brain Injury among Veterans," *Congressional Research Service*, January 4, 2013, www.ncbi.nlm.nih.gov/pubmed /22776913.

8. Denise Mann, "Bob Woodruff after Traumatic Brain Injury," WebMD, www.webmd.com/brain/features/bob-woodruff-after-traumatic-brain -injury, accessed February 6, 2016.

9. The wars in Iraq and Afghanistan took a record toll on journalists with more dying than in any other war since World War II. See Frank Smyth, "Iraq War and News Media: A Look Inside the Death Toll," Committee to Protect Journalists, https://cpj.org/blog/2013/03/iraq-war-and

-news-media-a-look-inside-the-death-to.php, accessed February 5, 2016. Smyth states that "at least 150 journalists and 54 media support workers" were killed in Iraq from March 2003 to December 2011, and at least 92 of them were "murdered in targeted assassinations."

10. Scott A. Marshall et al., "Traumatic Brain Injury," in *Combat Casualty Care: Lessons Learned from OEF and OIF*, edited by E. Savitsky and B. Eastridge (Falls Church, VA: Office of the Surgeon General, U.S. Army, 2012), 347.

11. Bagalman, "Traumatic Brain Injury among Veterans," 3.

12. Anderson Cooper, *360 Degrees*, CNN.com, February 2, 2006, www .cnn.com/TRANSCRIPTs/0602/02/acd.02.html.

13. Woodruff and Woodruff, *In an Instant*, 32.

14. Nazer H. Qureshi, "Skull Fracture," Medscape, September 10, 2015, http://emedicine.medscape.com/article/248108-overview. This article states that in one study "ten times more force was required to fracture a cadaveric skull with overlaying scalp than the one without."

15. Marshall et al., "Traumatic Brain Injury," 349.

16. Photographs and video of the Critical Care Transport Team are available at Donna Miles, "Air Guard Assists Critical Care Evacuations," U.S. Department of Defense, http://archive.defense.gov/news/newsarticle .aspx?id=63789, accessed February 5, 2016.

17. "Landstuhl Regional Medical Center," Army Medicine, www.goarmy .com/amedd/health-care/facilities/landstuhl-regional-medical-center .html, accessed February 5, 2016.

18. "Gabrielle Giffords' Extraordinary Journey," http://tirr .memorialhermann.org/patient-stories/gabrielle-giffords%e2%80 %99-extraordinary-journey/, accessed February 5, 2016. Abby Terrell, email to author, August 10, 2015.

19. Curtis Brainard, "Giffords' Medical Care: Healthy Dose of Science Coverage Adds Context," *Columbia Journalism Review*, January 12, 2011, www.cjr.org/the_observatory/giffords_medical_care.php; Sanjay Gupta, "Gupta: What Helped Giffords Survive Brain Shot," CNN.com, January 10, 2011, http://the chart.blogs.cnn.com/2011/01/10/gupta-how-giffords -survived-bullet-to-the-brain/.

20. "The Anatomy of the Brain," Mayfield Brain and Spine, www .mayfieldclinic.com/PE-AnatBrain.htm#.vcphm51VhHw, accessed September 1, 2015.

21. David Brown, "Giffords' Recovery Hinges on Brain Plasticity," *CBS News / Washington Post*, January 21, 2011, www.cbsnews.com/news /giffords-recovery-hinges-on-brain-plasticity/.

22. Ibid.

23. Norman Doidge, "Our Amazingly Plastic Brains," *Wall Street Journal*, February 6, 2015, www.wsj.com/articles/our-amazingly-plastic-brains-1423262095.

24. Ibid.

25. Brown, "Giffords' Recovery."

26. Woodruff and Woodruff, *In an Instant*, 147.

27. Alisa D. Gean, *Brain Injury: Applications from War and Terrorism* (Philadelphia: Lippincott, Williams and Wilkins, 2014), 11–15.

28. Lizette Alvarez, "War Veterans' Concussions Are Often Overlooked," *New York Times*, August 26, 2008, www.nytimes.com/2008/08/26.us/26tbi.html.

29. Ibid.

30. Ibid.

31. Ibid.

32. Bagalman, "Traumatic Brain Injury among Veterans," 3.

33. Bob Woodruff, "Gabrielle Giffords: Recovery from Brain Injury," *ABC News*, January 10, 2011, http://abcnews.go.com/Health/bob-woodruff-gabrielle-giffords-recover-brain-injury/story?id=12578057.

34. "To Iraq and Back: Bob Woodruff Reports," *ABC News*, February 2007, http://abcnews.go.com/Us/video/iraq-back-bob-woodruff-reports-5557859.

35. Woodruff and Woodruff, *In an Instant*, 255, 278, and passim.

36. Woodruff, "Gabrielle Giffords."

37. "Gabby Giffords Speaks Years into Her Recovery" (an interview with Lee Cowan), *CBS Sunday Morning*, March 15, 2015, www.cbsnews.com/videos/gabby-giffords-speaks-four-years-into-her-recovery/.

38. Woodruff, "Gabrielle Giffords."

12. THE TRAUMA WITHIN

1. "Phillips Petroleum Chemical Plant Explosion and Fire, Pasadena, Texas," US Fire Administration/Technical Report Series, USFA-TR-035/October 1989, FEMA, www.usfa.fema.gov/downloads/pdf/publications/tr-035.pdf.

2. The resulting blast measured 3.5 on the Richter scale twenty-five miles away and was later estimated to be 4.0 at the plant. Windows were blown out of a grade school two miles away. Debris from the plant was found as far as six miles from the blast.

3. Richard D. Allen, ed., *Handbook of Post Disaster Interventions*, special issue of *Journal of Social Behavior and Personality* 8 (1993): 287.

4. Bill Disessa, "Oct. 23, 1989: Terror from Phillips Blast Still Haunts," *Houston Chronicle*, October 21, 1990, www.chron.com/news/article/Oct-23 -1989-Terror-from-Phillips-blast-still-1486948.php.

5. Post-Traumatic Stress Disorder is defined as a mental health condition that is triggered by a terrifying event: "Post-Traumatic Stress Disorder," Mayo Clinic, http://www.mayoclinic.org/diseases-conditions /post-traumatic-stress-disorder/basics/definition/con-20022540, accessed February 5, 2015.

6. Allen, *Handbook of Post Disaster Interventions*, 290.

7. Ibid., 294.

8. Karen Krakower, "Compassion Fatigue: When You've Got Nothing Left to Give," *Health Leader*, University of Texas Health Science Center at Houston, November 15, 2005, www.westga.edu/~vickir/MentalHealth /MH16%20SecondaryStress/Secondary%20Stress%20Compassion %20Fatigue.pdf.

9. Matthew J. Friedman, "PTSD History and Overview," PTSD: National Center for PTSD, U.S. Department of Veterans Affairs, www.ptsd.va.gov /professional/PTSD-overview.asp, accessed October 1, 2015.

10. Kate Carlton Greer, "20 Years Later Oklahoma City Bombing Victims Fight Stigmas," *Weekend Edition Saturday*, NPR, April 19, 2015, www.npr .org/2015/04/18/400573585/20-years-later-oklahoma-city-bombing -victims-fight-stigmas.

11. Anemona Hartocollis, "10 Years and a Diagnosis Later, 9/11 Still Haunts," *New York Times*, August 9, 2011, www.nytimes.com/2011/08/10 /nyregion/post-traumatic-stress-disorder-from-911still-haunts.html?_r=0.

12. Robert Preidt, "Katrina Victims 10 Times More Prone to Post-Traumatic Stress," *ABC News*, May 18, 2007, http://abcnews.go.com /Health/Healthday/story?id=4507165&page=1.

13. Tony Horwitz, "Did Civil War Soldiers Have PTSD?," *Smithsonian*, January 2015, www.smithsonianmag.com/history/ptsd-civil-wars-hidden -legacy-180953652/.

14. Paula Span, "No End to Trauma for Some Older Veterans," *New York Times*, March 15, 2013, http://newoldage.blogs.nytimes.com/2013/03/15 /no-end-to-trauma-for-some-older-veterans/. Span notes that some World War II veterans ignored signs of PTSD until they were retired and then were overcome by symptoms after retirement or even in their eighties.

15. David J. Morris, *The Evil Hours: A Biography of Post-Traumatic Stress Disorder* (New York: Houghton Mifflin, 2015), 139.

16. *Born on the Fourth of July* was written by Ron Kovic, a former marine

from a small town who was paralyzed from the chest down by a bullet during the Vietnam War. See Steve Lopez, "Forty Years after 'Fourth of July' Ron Kovic Still Speaking Up against War," *Los Angeles Times*, November 8, 2014, http://www.latimes.com/local/california/la-me-1109-lopez-kovic-20141109-column.html.

17. Morris, *The Evil Hours*,141.

18. Ibid., 147.

19. Ibid., 156.

20. The National Center for PTSD, www.ptsd.va.gov/, accessed October 1, 2015.

21. C. W. Hoge et al., "Combat Duty in Iraq and Afghanistan, Mental Health Problems, and Barriers to Care," *New England Journal of Medicine* 351 (2004): 13–21.

22. Leo Shane III, "Retirement Might Unleash PTSD Symptoms in Vietnam Veterans," *Stars and Stripes*, June 20, 2012, www.stripes.com/news/retirement-might-unleash-ptsd-symptoms-in-vietnam-veterans-1.180888.

23. Ibid.

24. Ibid.

25. "A New Therapy for a New Generation: An Interview with Albert 'Skip' Rizzo," *Frontline*, PBS.org, March 24, 2009, www.pbs.org/wgbh/pages/frontline/digitalnation/extras/interviews/rizzo.html.

26. Jeffrey Kluger, "The 2010 Time 100: Edna Foa," *Time*, April 29, 2010, http://content.time.com/time/specials/packages/article/0,28804,1984685_1984745_1985506,00.html.

27. Eleanor Beardsley, "70 Years On, a Normandy Village Honors Aging WWII Vets," *Morning Edition*, NPR.org, June 5, 2014, www.npr.org/sections/parallels/2014/06/05/319030313/70-years-on-a-normandy-village-honors-aging-wwii-veterans.

28. Rob McIlvaine, "3-D Software Becoming Safeware to Returning Soldiers with PTSD," U.S. Army, January 28, 2011, www.army.mil/article/51066/3_D_software_becoming_safeware_to_returning_Soldiers_with_PTSD/.

29. "A New Therapy for a New Generation: An Interview with Albert 'Skip' Rizzo."

30. G. M. Reger et al., "Effectiveness of Virtual Reality Exposure Therapy for Active Duty Soldiers in a Military Mental Health Clinic," *Journal of Traumatic Stress* 24 (February 2011): 95.

31. David J. Morris, "After PTSD, More Trauma," *New York Times*,

January 17, 2015, http://opinionator.blogs.nytimes.com/2015/01/17/after
-ptsd-more-trauma/#more-155563.

32. John Galen Buckwalter, "Stress Resilience in Virtual Environments
(STRIVE)," Instituted for Creative Technologies USC, http://ict.usc.edu
/prototypes/strive/, accessed October 1, 2015.

33. Jan Hoffman, "Nightmares after the ICU," *New York Times*, July 22,
2013, http://well.blogs.nytimes.com/2013/07/22/nightmares-after-the
-i-c-u/?_r=0.

34. Nancy Andrews, "Delirious," www.nancyandrews.net/section
/delirious, accessed February 5, 2016. Andrews give a riveting first-person
account of her experiences in the ICU and after. Her website also includes
an information resource page for post-ICU PTSD.

35. Daniela J. Lamas, "Flashbacks Plague Former ICU Patients," *Boston
Globe*, April 8, 2013, https://www.bostonglobe.com/lifestyle/health
-wellness/2013/04/07/delirium-induced-flashbacks-plague-many
-former-icu-patients/a7547VfsYc8rWDjG1NDkIj/story.html.

36. Sarah Wake and Deborah Kitchiner, "Post-traumatic Stress Disorder
after Intensive Care," *British Medical Journal* 346 (2013), www.bmj.com
/content/346/bmj.f3232.

37. Ibid.

38. D. S. Davydow, J. M. Gifford, S. V. Desai, D. M. Needham, and O. J.
Bienvenu, "Posttraumatic Stress Disorder in General Intensive Care Unit
Survivors: A Systematic Review," *General Hospital Psychiatry* 30 (2008): 426.

39. Ed Susman, "PTSD Common Following ICU Stay," MedpageToday.
com, May 21, 2014, www.medpagetoday.com/MeetingCoverage/ATS
/45904.

40. Ibid.

41. Rick Nauert, "Hospital Diaries Protect from PTSD," *Psych Central
News*, September 17, 2010, http://psychcentral.com/news/2010/09/17
/hospital-diaries-protect-from-ptsd/18334.html.

42. Lois Beckett, "Why Hospitals Are Failing Civilians Who Get PTSD,"
ProPublica, March 4, 2014, www.propublica.org/article/why-hospitals-are
-failing-civilians-who-get-ptsd#.

43. Ibid.

44. Ibid.

45. Deborah A. Hood, "PTSD in Nurses," Advance Healthcare Network:
Advances for Nurses, February 4, 2011, http://nursing.advanceweb.com
/Features/Articles/PTSD-in-Nurses.aspx.

46. Fran Lowry, "Emergency Department Staff Not Immune to Trau-

matic Stress," March 5, 2015, Medscape.com, www.medscape.com
/viewarticle/840980.

47. Ibid.

48. Ibid.

49. Judith Graham, "For Some Caregivers, the Trauma Lingers," *New York Times*, January 30, 2013, http://newoldage.blogs.nytimes.com/2013
/01/30/for-some-caregivers-the-trauma-lingers/?_r=0.

50. Judith Graham, "After the Caregiving Ends," *New York Times*, March 7, 2013, http://newoldage.blogs.nytimes.com/2013/03/07/after-the
-caregiving-ends/.

51. Ibid.

52. Yvette Orozco, "20 Years Later," *Your Houston News*, October 25, 2009, www.yourhoustonnews.com/deer_park/news/years-later/article
_ab14633b-1c5e-51c7-a344-c88b238838c0.html.

13. THE ROAD BACK

1. Stanley Yoo, "From Doctor to Patient," *The Cord*, Jefferson and Magee Regional Spinal cord Injury Cord Center of the Delaware Valley, www
.spinalcordcenter.org/consumer/pdf-files/cordspring2009.pdf., accessed November 1, 2015.

2. "Steve Shope's Story," Trail to Recovery, www.trailtorecovery.com
/index.php/our-story, accessed November 3, 2016.

3. Cervical spinal cord injury can occur from level C1 to C8 and is characterized by paralysis of both arms and legs and loss of bowel, bladder, and sexual function. Thoracic spinal cord injury, T1 to T12, is less common because of protection afforded the thoracic spine by the rib cage and usually involves the lower extremities as well as bowel, bladder, and sexual function. Lumbar spinal cord injury, L1 to L5, affects the legs and pelvic organs. Sacral spinal cord injury, S1 to S5, involves the pelvic organs. A spinal cord injury is also classified as complete—that is, all the function below a certain level is affected—versus incomplete, where some messages between brain and spinal cord are still able to get through. "Spinal Cord Injury Types," Spinal Cord Injury-Paralysis Resource Center, Christopher and Dana Reeves Foundation, www.christopherreeve.org/site/c
.mtKZKgMWKwg/b.4514603/k.77E9/Spinal_Cord_Injury_Types.htm, accessed November 3, 2015.

4. Mark G. Burnett and Eric L. Zager, "Pathophysiology of Peripheral Nerve Injury: A Brief Review," *Medscape General Surgery*, www.medscape
.com/viewarticle/480071_5, accessed February 5, 2016.

5. "Emergency Management: What Immediate Procedures Can I Expect," Dana and Christopher Reeve Foundation, www.christopherreeve.org/site/c.mtKZKgMWKwg/b.4514601/k.6A58/Emergency_management.htm, accessed November 3, 2015.

6. This is a computer analogy: CPU means "central processing unit."

7. "Spinal Cord Injury Facts and Figures at a Glance," February 2012, National Spinal Cord Injury Statistical Center, Birmingham, Alabama, https://www.nscisc.uab.edu.

8. Eric Pace, "Howard Rusk, 88, Dies; Medical Pioneer," *New York Times*, November 5, 1989.

9. Howard A. Rusk, *A World to Care For: The Autobiography of Howard A. Rusk MD* (New York: Random House, 1972), 56.

10. "Howard A. Rusk (1901–1989)," State Historical Society of Missouri: Historic Missourians, http://shs.umsystem.edu/historicmissourians/name/r/rusk/index.html, accessed November 1, 2015.

11. Timothy R. Dillingham, "Physiatry, Physical Medicine, and Rehabilitation: Historical Development and Military Roles," *Physical Medicine and Rehabilitation Clinics of North America* 13 (February 2002): 3.

12. C. George Kevorkian, Matthe Bartels, and Deborah J. Franklin, "To Believe in Humanity and Rehabilitation: Howard A. Rusk, MD, and the Birth of Rehabilitation Medicine," *Physical Medicine and Rehabilitation* 5 (April 2013): 248.

13. Rusk, *A World to Care For*, 65.

14. Ibid., 56.

15. Ibid., 98.

16. Ibid., 100.

17. Ibid., 249.

18. "Biographical Sketch," Howard A. Rusk Papers, http://shs.umsystem.edu/manuscripts/invent/3981.pdf. accessed November 1, 2015.

19. Nava Blum and Elizabeth Fee, "Howard A. Rusk (1901–1989): From Military Medicine to Comprehensive Rehabilitation," *American Journal of Public Health* 98 (2008): 256–57.

20. Pace, "Howard Rusk."

21. Kevorkian, Bartels, and Franklin, "To Believe in Humanity and Rehabilitation," 248.

22. Blum and Fee, "Howard A. Rusk."

23. Pace, "Howard Rusk."

24. Howard A. Rusk, *A World to Care For: The Autobiography of Howard A. Rusk MD* (New York: Random House, 1972), 181.

25. "How Locomotor Training Works," Christopher and Dana Reeve Foundation, www.christopherreeve.org/site/c.ddJFKRNoFig/b.5399935/k .e273/How_Locomotor_Training_works.htm, accessed October 15, 2015. See also "What Is Locomotor Training," YouTube video, https://www .youtube.com/watch?v=gTQ5PdF_YR8, accessed October 15, 2016.

26. "Locomotor Training at Magee Rehabilitation Hospital," YouTube video, https://www.youtube.com/watch?v=x_EVNaOMChU, accessed November 6, 2015.

27. Stanley Yoo, "From Doctor to Patient," *The Cord*, Jefferson and Magee Regional Spinal Cord Injury Cord Center of the Delaware Valley, www.spinalcordcenter.org/consumer/pdf-files/cordspring2009.pdf., accessed November 1, 2015.

28. "Steve Shope's Story," Trail to Recovery, www.trailtorecovery.com /index.php/our-story, accessed November 3, 3015.

29. Wise Young, "Life Expectancy after Spinal Cord Injury," Care Cure Community, June 1, 2012, http://sci.rutgers.edu/forum/showthread.php ?189092-Life-Expectancy-after-Spinal-Cord-Injury.

30. John W. McDonald, "Repairing the Damaged Spinal Cord," *Scientific American*, November 6, 2008, www.scientificamerican.com/article /repairing-the-damaged-spinal-cord/.

31. Rachel Kessler, "Neuro-Spinal Scaffold for Repair of Spinal Cord Injuries: Interview with InVivo CEO," *Medgadget*, September 25, 2015, www .medgadget.com/2015/09/neuro-spinal-scaffold-repair-spinal-cord -injuries-interview-invivo-ceo.html.

32. Adario Strange, "FDA Approves First Robotic Exoskeleton for Paralyzed Users," *Mashable*, June 30, 2014, http://mashable.com/2014/06/30 /fda-approves-robotic-exoskeleton-paralyzed-rewalk/#lWdARCB3lgq3.

33. Christina Jakubowski, "The Future of Treatments for Spinal Cord Injury," *Bioscience Technology*, December 2, 2014, www.biosciencetechnology .com/articles/2014/12/future-treatments-spinal-cord-injury.

34. "From Spinal Injury Patient to CrossFit Champ," PHIL17, November 13, 2013, http://phl17.com/2013/11/13/from-spinal-injury-patient-to -crossfit-champ/; CrossFit 215, November 8, 2012, https://www.facebook .com/CrossFit215/posts/462317470478211.

14. LOSING A LIMB, FINDING A CAUSE

1. Cory Tomesh, "The Mike Schultz Story," ESPN.com, April 8, 2009, http://espn.go.com/action/news/story?id=4052161.

2. Ibid.

3. Peter Maguire and Colin Murray Parkes, "Surgery and Loss of Body Parts," *British Medical Journal* 316 (April 4, 1998): 1086.

4. Wayne Drehs, "Mike Schultz: Life Is about Adapting," ESPN.com, January 27, 2013, http://xgames.espn.go.com/xgames/rally-moto-x /article/8883736/adaptive-snocross-racer-mike-schultz-lost-leg-lose-drive.

5. Drehs, "Mike Schultz."

6. John Nosta, "The Amazing Saga of Mike Schultz, Citizen Scientist," *Forbes*, September 27, 2013, www.forbes.com/sites/johnnosta/2013/09/27 /the-amazing-saga-of-mike-schultz-citizen-scientist/.

7. Christine Miller, "Battlefield Injuries: Saving Lives and Limbs throughout History," *Lower Extremity Review Magazine*, October 2013, http://lermagazine.com/cover_story/battlefield-injuries-saving-lives-and -limbs-throughout-history.

8. Hannah Fischer, "A Guide to U.S. Military Casualty Statistics: Operation Freedom's Sentinel, Operation Inherent Resolve, Operation New Dawn, Operation Iraqi Freedom, and Operation Enduring Freedom," Congressional Research Service, August 7, 2015, https://www.fas.org/sgp /crs/natsec/RS22452.pdf, p. 6. This article defines major limb amputation as "the loss of one or more limbs, the loss of one or more partial limbs, or the loss of one or more full or partial hand or foot."

9. Miller, "Battlefield Injuries."

10. Steve Almasy, "The Toll of War Now Includes More Amputees," CNN.com, October 29, 2012, www.cnn.com/2012/05/27/us/amputee -veterans-come-home/.

11. Miller, "Battlefield Injuries."

12. "iWalk BiOM, Medical Center Orthotics and Prosthetics," https:// mcopro.com/cptechnology/iwalk-biom/, accessed November 1, 2015.

13. Chris Higgins, "Antlers Inspire First Trial of Bone-Implanted Pros- thetics," *Wired*, September 9, 2014, www.wired.co.uk/news/archive/2014 -09/09/prosthetic-legs-attached-to-bone.

14. Paul F. Pasquina and Rory A. Cooper, *Care of the Combat Amputee* (Falls Church, VA: Office of the Surgeon General, U.S. Army, 2009), 723, https://ke.army.mil/bordeninstitute/published_volumes/amputee /CCAchapter27.pdf.

15. Chuck Seegert, "Antler-Inspired Prosthesis Breaches Skin Barrier," *Med Device Online*, September 11, 2014, www.meddeviceonline.com/doc /antler-inspired-prosthesis-breaches-skin-barrier-0001.

16. Stav Ziv, "Mind-Controlled Prosthetic Arm Tested in Sweden," *News-*

week, October 8, 2014, www.newsweek.com/mind-controlled-prosthetic
-arm-tested-sweden-276281.

17. Ibid.

18. "A Blueprint for Restoring Touch with a Prosthetic Hand," University
of Chicago Medicine, October 14, 2013, www.uchospitals.edu/news/2013
/20131014-prosthetic-hand.html.

19. Marty McKee, "The Six Million Dollar Man: Plot Summary," *IMDB*,
www.imdb.com/title/tt0071054/plotsummary?ref_=tt_stry_pl.

20. Linda Carroll, "Double Arm Transplant Vet 'Getting a Second
Chance,'" *NBC News*, January 29, 2013, www.nbcnews.com/id/50628032
/ns/health-mens_health/t/double-arm-transplant-soldier-getting
-second-chance/.

21. "Soldier Gets Double-Arm Transplant at Johns Hopkins," Associated
Press, January 28, 2013, http://www.usatoday.com/story/news/nation
/2013/01/28/double-arm-transplant-soldier/1870357/.

22. Michael E. Ruane, "With Transplanted Arms and Army Grit, a
Quadruple Amputee Soldiers On," *Washington Post*, June 30, 2014, www
.washingtonpost.com/local/with-transplanted-arms-and-army-grit-a
-quadruple-amputee-soldiers-on/2014/06/30/5130c242-f6e8-11e3-a3a5
-42be35962a52_story.html.

23. Keith Deutsch, *Operation Rebound*, "Frontline to Finish Line,"
www.challengedathletes.org/atf/cf/%7B10E89006-A432-401E-BC75
-805E68CE5C27%7d/DEUTSCH,k..pDF, accessed February 6, 2016, see
also *The Hero's Project*, "U.S. Army Sargent Retired Keith Deutsch," http://
theheroesproject.org/people/us-army-sgt-retired-keith-deutsch/, accessed
February 6, 2016.

24. X Games Aspen, "Mike Schultz's Connection to Veteran's Day"
(video), http://xgames.espn.go.com/xgames/video/14104283/mike
-schultz-connection-veterans-day, accessed February 6, 2016.

25. Mike Schultz, "Restoration," *Player's Tribune*, November 11, 2015,
www.theplayerstribune.com/mike-schultz-biodapt-prosthetics/.

INDEX

Note: page numbers followed by n refer to notes, with note number.

40; as research mentor, 42-44; research on airplane accidents, 41-42; research on injury cause and prevention, 2, 30-33, 35-37, 39, 40-41

Banks, Sam, 66

Baruch, Bernard, 191

battle fatigue, 171

battlefield injuries: advances in gun technology and, 24-25, 141; exsanguination as leading cause of death in, 94

battlefield injuries, treatment of: case study, 94, 96-98; MARCH protocol for, 95; prioritization of bleeding in, 95. *See also* war

Bell UH-1 Iroquois ("Huey") helicopter, 53-57, 58

Billings, Frank, 189

Bioadapt Co., 206

Blaisdell, William, 86

Blalock, Alfred, 78-79

bleeding, stopping of: case study, 94, 96-98; experience of, described, 92-93; in gunshot victims, 109-10; prioritization of in trauma care, 95; technology for, 96; tourniquets and, 95-96

bleeding out (exsanguination): as common cause of trauma death, 93-94; percentage of preventable deaths from, 94-95

blood, artificial, 104-5

blood bank system: development of, 21, 98-100; increasing demands on, 98, 105; reliance of donations, 98; and safety of blood supply, 104; standardization of collection techniques, 100

Blood for Britain project, 100

bloodmobiles, 100

blood pharming, 105

Blood Transfusion Betterment Association, 99

Boston Marathon bombings, 2

box jellyfish, stings of, 129-30, 133, 134

brain: adaptability after damage (neuroplasticity), 160-61; areas controlling specific functions in, 159-60; function, severe cold and, 126. *See also* traumatic brain injury (TBI)

Brown, Mitchell, 62, 63, 73

burn injuries, 43, 137-38

Cambridge Military Hospital (England), facial injury ward at, 142-43

cardiac arrest: ambulance services of 1960s and, 62-63, 65; and development of portable defibrillator, 68-69

cardiac units, mobile, development of, 70-71

Caroline, Nancy, 68, 71

Catalan, Max Ortiz, 205

Christopher and Dana Reeve Foundation, 193, 195, 197

Civil Rights Act of 1964, 64

Civil War: casualties in, 21; collection of trauma data in, 26-27; crude medical/surgical methods in, 22, 23, 25-26; development of modern Army medical corps, 27-29; early lack of system for care of wounded, 20, 21-22, 23, 24, 26; new weapons, increased

to reduce, 147, 148; skin grafts and, 142, 145–47, 149

as cause of deaths, 94; causes of, 153; incidence in U.S., 153; in Iraq and Afghanistan wars, 151–53, 154, 156, 157, 161–65, 166; long-term effects of, 163–64; rating severity of, 153, 162; soldiers' increasing survival of, 152; swelling in, 154–55, 157, 158, 159, 162; treatment of, 154, 155–56, 157, 159, 165, 166, 174; underdiagnosis of, 163
tube pedicle flaps, 146–47

Valadier, Auguste, 141–42, 147
Veterans Administration (VA), 172, 173, 190
Vietnam War: and antiwar movement, 171, 172; helicopter ambulances in, 53–57; medical advances in, 21, 24, 85–86; medics in, 71; and PTSD, 171–72, 173–74, 175
virtual reality exposure therapy, 174–77
Voting Rights Act of 1962, 64

war: and helicopter ambulances, 49–57; lessons in trauma care from, 2, 8, 20; new medical challenges of each, 21, 23–24. *See also specific wars*
Weathers, Beck, 124–28
Webster, Daniel, 115–16
Whitman, Charles, 106–7, 108, 110–11, 117
"Whole Person" concept, 191–92

wilderness injuries: definition of, 120; in national parks, 131–33; wide range of, 128, 131
wilderness medicine: case studies, 119, 127–28, 128–30, 131; courses in, 121, 130; and evacuation of injured, 120, 128; increasing need for, 119–20, 121–22; and medical supplies, 120, 122–23, 130–31; origins of, 120–21; physicians in, 121, 122–23
Wilson, Claire, 106–7, 108, 117
Winston, Flaura, 42–43
Woodruff, Bob, 151–53, 154, 156, 157, 161–62, 164–65, 166
World War I: and development of plastic surgery, 21, 141–47, 149–50; head and neck wounds in, 23–24, 140–41; limitations of medical treatment in, 141, 190; number of casualties in, 140; and PTSD, 171; and rehabilitation medicine, 189
World War II: and blood bank system, 98–100; helicopter ambulances in, 49–57; medical advances in, 21; paraplegic soldiers, life expectancy of, 190; and PTSD, 171; and rehabilitation medicine, 188–90; and wilderness medicine, development of, 120–21

XStat device, 96

Yoo, Stanley, 185, 192–94, 196–97